Attention Deficit-Hyperactivity Disorder

H. Moghadam, MD

and Colleagues

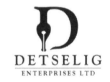

DETSELIG
ENTERPRISES LTD

Calgary, Alberta

Attention Deficit-Hyperactivity Disorder

National Library of Canada Cataloguing in Publication

Moghadam, H. (Hossein)
    Attention deficit-hyperactivity disorder / H. Moghadam.

Includes bibliographical references.
ISBN-13: 978-1-55059-309-9
ISBN-10: 1-55059-309-9

1. Attention-deficit hyperactivity disorder. I, Title.

RJ506.H9M64 2006   618.92'8589   C2006-901695-X

Detselig Enterprises Ltd.   Phone: (403) 283-0900
210 - 1220 Kensington Rd. SW   Fax: (403) 283-6947
Calgary, Alberta T2N 3P5   Email: temeron@telusplanet.net
                                 www.temerondetselig.com

We acknowledge the support of the Government of Canada through the Book Publishing Industry Development Program (BPIDP) for our publishing program.
We also acknowledge the support of the Alberta Foundation for the Arts for our publishing program.

SAN: 113-0234   Printed in Canada

Cover Design by Alvin Choong
Illustrations by Heather Sawyer

*This book is dedicated to all misunderstood
children, their parents and teachers.*

Disclaimer

This book is a concise source of information on attention deficit-hyperactivity disorder and, as such, does not attempt to completely cover this complex topic. It discusses the principal aspects of what is currently known about it but the brevity of the presentation precludes detailed discussions. The book is not intended to be a substitute for your physician's advice. Every child with ADHD is a unique individual and his/her management should be individually designed in keeping with the particular circumstances of the child, the family, and the classroom teacher. Neither the authors, nor the publisher, accept any legal or moral responsibility, or any liability, for actions taken by parents that are contrary to the advice of their family physician.

Brand names of medications have been included in the book because, normally, parents and teachers are not familiar with drugs' generic names. This is not to be construed, however, as an endorsement or a criticism of these or other products. Statements regarding the therapeutic properties, the effectiveness, and the side effects of the drugs mentioned in this book are based entirely on the authors' experience and may differ from the experience of other physicians.

Authors

Primary Author

H. Moghadam, MD, MPH, FRCPC
Emeritus Professor of Pediatrics and Community
Health Sciences, University of Calgary.

Contributing Authors

Samuel y-y Chang, MD, FRCPC
Child and adolescent Psychiatrist
Clinical Associate Professor, Department of Psychiatry,
University of Calgary.

**Geraldine Farrelly, LRCP,LRCS, DCH (Irel),
D.Obst, FRCPC**
Developmental Pediatrician, Clinical Associate
Professor, Departments of Pediatrics and Psychiatry,
University of Calgary

Thiru Govender, MD, FRCPC
Developmental Pediatrician, Clinical Associate
Professor,
Department of Pediatrics, University of Calgary

Stephen Maunula, MSc
Psychologist, Alberta Children's Hospital

Carol Skelly, MEd
Education Consultant, Alberta Children's Hospital

Mila Wendt, MSW
Social Worker, Alberta Children's Hospital

Acknowledgments

The authors wish to thank the following people who reviewed various parts of this book and provided many practical comments and helpful suggestions:

Debbie and Raymond Abry, Alexa Nemberg, Fiorenza Russel, Roberta Travis, all parents of ADHD children; Dr. Valerie Barsky, psychologist, Mental Health Services, Calgary Health Region; Dr. Juanne Clarke, professor of sociology, Wilfrid Laurier University, Kitchener, Ontario; Alanna Edwards, M.Ed. faculty member, Media Studies Department, Malaspina University College, Nanaimo, British Columbia; Dr. Bonnie J. Kaplan, Professor of Pediatrics and Community Health Sciences, University of Calgary; Susan J. Maunula, psychologist, Calgary Learning Centre; Dr. Ross McDonald, family physician, Calgary, Alberta, and Gaynor Strobel, teacher-librarian, Shawnigan Lake School, Vancouver Island, British Columbia.

The tolerance and patience of Kris Webber-Shushkewich and Jill Sugars during the preparation of the manuscript are greatly appreciated.

We are also grateful to Heather Sawyer for the illustrations in this book.

Table of Contents

Preface

The first version of this book, *Attention Deficit Disorder*, was published in 1988 when there was very little published material available for parents and teachers of children with attention deficit-hyperactivity disorder. The topic was controversial and most people, including many professionals, questioned its very existence. Since then ADHD has become widely accepted as a disabling deviation from normal mental processes that affects a significant segment of the population of all ages. Despite this widespread acceptance, many children affected by this disorder continue to underachieve academically, and to experience conflict and disappointments in their personal relationships. It is the authors' hope that this book will help those experiencing such difficulties, as well as their caregivers, to attain a higher quality of life. While in the following pages we address ADHD in children and adolescents, it is important to know that most, but not all, of the affected individuals continue having problems throughout their lives. For the interested adult with ADHD, we have included a list of additional sources of information at the end of this book.

ADHD is a common problem affecting at least one or two children in every classroom in North America. The impetus for writing the first version of this book was provided by the parents and teachers of children attending the clinics of the Alberta Children's Hospital where children with ADHD were evaluated and treated. They often wanted a concise source of information on this perplexing problem and the rationale for the recommended approaches to its management. Neither the previous nor the current version of this book has been intended to be a scientific discourse or the final word on ADHD. Rather, our intention has been to supply the readers with sufficient information to enable them to make informed treatment decisions. Instead of making references to scientific journals that would be of little value to most readers, we provide a list of additional readings and websites.

Attention Deficit-Hyperactivity Disorder has been prepared with major contributions by the professional staff of the Child Health and Mental Health Programs of the Calgary Health Region and the Calgary Learning Centre. Throughout this book male gender has been used for the sake of simplicity. The disorder affects both males and females.

1   A Brief Historical Review

Our youth now loves luxury. They have bad manners, contempt for authority and disrespect for their elders. Children nowadays are tyrants.

Socrates, 470-399 BC

Attention Deficit/ Hyperactivity Disorder has been most likely around since ancient times.

The earliest known description of hyperactive behaviour in a child was, however, provided in a children's storybook, published in 1845 by a German physician, Dr. Heinrich Hoffmann. In that book, *Der Struwwelpeter* (Unkempt Peter), there is a particular story of interest, "Die Geschichte vom Zappel Philipp" (the story of fidgety Phil). Some readers may be familiar with various translations that have retained its original style of doggerel verse. The first few lines of one translation are as follows:

> Phil, stop acting like a worm
> The table is not a place to squirm.
> Thus speaks the father to his son
> Severely says it, not in fun.
> Mother frowns and looks around
> Although she doesn't make a sound.
> But Philipp will not take advice,
> He'll have his way at any price.
> He turns,
> And churns.
> He wiggles
> And jiggles
> Here and there on the chair.
> Phil, these twists I can not bear.

"Der Struwwelpeter (Unkempt Peter)

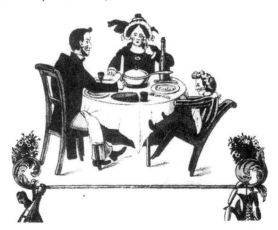

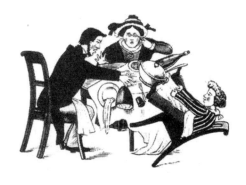

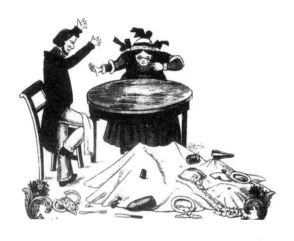

Some decades later, in 1902, a distinguished British pediatrician, Dr. George F. Still, made reference to misbehaving children who were refractory to discipline. Whether these children were exhibiting the manifestations of ADHD or other types of maladaptive behaviour is not clear.

Nothing else appeared in the literature until the third decade of the 20th century. Toward the end of the World War 1 many countries experienced an epidemic of brain infection (encephalitis), often associated with severe lethargy (sleep sickness or Von Economo's encephalitis lethargica). Many of the adults who survived the acute illness subsequently developed a disorder known as Parkinson's syndrome which consisted of various degrees of muscle rigidity, an abnormal gait, shaky arms and hands, expressionless face, drooling, and disturbances of attention, memory and emotion. On the other hand, some of the children who survived the acute illness developed a constellation of behavioral traits similar to what we now know as attention deficit-hyperactivity disorder. This is the origin of the now discredited *minimal brain damage*. It was, however, soon realized that there were also many children with similar constellation of behavioral traits who had not suffered from encephalitis or any other type of frank brain damage. Over the years the label was replaced by *minimal brain dysfunction*, which still lingers in some popular writings.

In 1937, Dr. Charles A. Bradley, an American Psychiatrist, described a group of institutionalized emotionally disturbed children who responded to treatment with Benzedrine, a stimulant drug. They showed increased interest in schoolwork, better work habits and an improvement in their disruptive behaviour. This improvement, which ran contrary to intuition, could not be explained until several decades later when research on the functioning of the brain provided an understanding of this mystery.

In 1957, Ritalin (methylphenidate) was marketed for the treatment of hyperactive children. It was found effective for some of these children. In the 1960s and early 1970s there was a wave of over-prescribing stimulant drugs for the treatment of many types of problem behaviors and failure at school. This overuse (far less common today) led to a justifiable outcry by many teachers, other professionals, parents and even some physicians, against the practice of "medicating" children for their problem behaviors. These protests have led to a much more rational use of stimulant medications and have provided an impetus for vastly increased research into the causes and treatment of ADHD. Although much still remains to be learned about ADHD, we have now a far better understanding of this disorder and how stimulant drugs work to alleviate its symptoms. Based on the recent scientific discoveries, the National Institute of Health in the United States, recognized ADHD as a legitimate medical condition in 1998.

2   ADHD – What is It?

On every scientist's desk there is a drawer labeled "unknown" in which he files what are at the moment unsolved questions, lest through guesswork or impatient speculation he come upon incorrect answers that will do him more harm than good. Man's worst fault is opening the drawer too soon. His task is not to discover final answers but to win the best partial answers that he can, from which others may move confidently against the unknown, to win better ones.

Homer W. Smith, 1895-1962

It is ironic that an abundance of writings on any topic, whether in scientific journals or in popular press, is often an indication of our inadequate understanding of that topic. As an example consider poliomyelitis, a well-known disease with often disabling consequences. Most readers of this book have not seen an individual afflicted with this crippling condition but know that it is a disease that can be prevented through routine immunization of children. When we discovered the cause of poliomyelitis and learned how to prevent it, it was eradicated in most countries. It is no longer a threat to our health and, therefore, there is no interest in reading or writing about it. Neither in scientific journals nor in popular press does one find articles about poliomyelitis. Now consider cancer, a common and incompletely understood group of diseases. It is hardly possible to find a medical journal or a popular magazine without an article on cancer. Cancer is still a major threat to our health and we still have a great deal to learn about its various forms. As long as the search for cause and prevention goes on, scientist will publish the results of their investigations in professional journals. Some of these findings also seep into popular press.

Attention deficit-hyperactivity disorder belongs to this latter category. Between 1957 and 1960, less than three dozen articles appeared in the scientific journals on this topic;. twenty years later, between 1987 and 1990, over 7000 articles were published. The search for answers to this complex condition has continued relentlessly up to the present time, indicating that we still have a great deal to learn about it. There is even a newsletter, *ADHD Report*, published every two months, that attempts to keep professionals current with new developments in the field.

For many years this condition was the source of both interest and controversy among psychiatrists, neurologists, pediatricians, psychologists, educators and the general public. Some reputed scientists questioned its very existence. At times, this controversy reached the political arena when some concerned citizens attempted to influence the lawmakers to ban certain forms of its treatment. As a result of scientific discoveries of the past decade or so, there is no longer any question that this disabling condition affects a significant segment of the population of all ages and has important sociological and economic consequences for society as a whole. As is the case with many other conditions affecting the health and well-being of individuals, there are still some groups among the general population who question the validity of recent scientific discoveries which, incidentally, have also substantiated the rationale for the hitherto empirical treatment of ADHD.

The behavioral problems common to the children with ADHD will be discussed in details in later chapters. We now recognize different subtypes of this disorder, each subtype presenting a different predominant problem:

The predominant problem in one subtype that affects many ADHD children is an impairment of their ability to focus and sustain their attention on a task and to avoid distraction at a level appropriate for their age. They may or may not be noticeably hyperactive.

In other ADHD children, the predominant problems are: 1) hyperactivity; i.e., a difficulty to regulate their motor activities so that their movements are purposeful and goal-oriented and 2) impulsiveness which makes it difficult for them to resist immediate temptations and to modulate their behaviour consistent with their age. They may have varying degrees of inattention.

Still in other ADHD children, inattention, distractibility, impulsivity and hyperactivity, as well as other age-inappropriate behaviors, occur simultaneously.

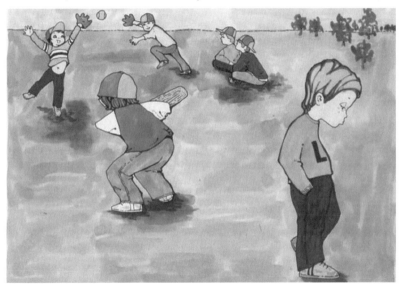

It is important to know that inattention can result from many causes. In this book we will discuss mainly the inattention that results from a developmental failure of certain areas of the brain which in turn leads to significant learning and social difficulties. There are, however, children whose inattention is caused by other factors. These include chaotic family circumstances, inappropriate expectations of the child by his parents or teachers and, occasionally, a conscious effort on the part of the child to avoid humiliation. Chronic insufficient sleep, inadequate or no breakfast, or being subject to frequent intimidations or beatings by bullies can all contribute to inattention in school. Sleep disorders such as snoring and sleep apnea (temporary cessation of breathing) can also lead to hyperactivity and inattention. Also, children with specific learning disabilities; i.e., children whose main difficulty is processing auditory and or visual information (spoken and written words) may become inattentive when they are confronted with the challenge of learning to read, write or do arithmetic. When the learning task becomes overwhelming for the learning-disabled child, his attention wanes, he becomes easily distracted and may become even somewhat fidgety. However, this behaviour is apparent only in academic settings. ADHD children are, on the other hand, inattentive in multiple settings: in school, at home, in church, on the playground, etc.

The inattention of children with ADHD is the result of an intrinsic deficiency of the brain circuitry that monitors inhibition and self-control. This inefficient self-regulation is a **neurological** disorder that impairs brain functions crucial for focused and sustained attention and is the principal cause of their difficulties. Some authorities refer to this as *primary inattention* as opposed to the type of inattention caused by other factors mentioned above.

There are, of course, children who experience a mixture of attention, learning, behavioral and emotional problems. For example, we know that many ADHD children also have other conditions such as mood disorders, anxiety, as well as disruptive behaviour disorders. These will be discussed in chapter 11.

It is thus apparent that when assessing a child with a possible diagnosis of ADHD, it is very important to obtain a highly detailed history from the parents and other caregivers of the child in order to establish an accurate diagnosis. Clearly, ADHD is a common and complex problem with significant academic, social and economic consequences for the affected individuals, their families and the society.

3   The Prevalence of ADHD

Truth in all its kind is most difficult to win; and truth in medicine is the most difficult of all

Peter mere Latham, 1789-1875

In the previous chapter we discussed inattention, impulsiveness and hyperactivity in ADHD children as behavioral traits inconsistent with their age. It must, however, be stated that we are neither sufficiently precise in our definitions nor have instruments that would accurately measure these behaviors. When two different rating scales (usually questionnaires) are used to identify hyperactive children, parents and teachers do not always pick out the same children, even if both questionnaires have been validated for their reliability on the normal childhood population. Similarly, children who are inattentive and easily distracted in the classroom can be seen totally absorbed in other activities at home such as watching a favorite television show. It is for this reason that measuring the prevalence of ADHD has proved a difficult task and has remained an approximation at best. The American Psychiatric Association has attempted to devise diagnostic criteria for ADHD in order to differentiate it from other disruptive behaviors of childhood. The first attempt was made in 1968 in the second edition of the *Diagnostic and Statistical Manual* or DSM II for short. In subsequent editions in 1980, 1987, 1994 and 2000, revisions to these criteria were made. The diagnostic criteria in the last revision of the DSM will be presented in chapter 5.

The published studies of the prevalence of ADHD have not always used the above diagnostic criteria. Nor is it always clear that when used, how strictly the criteria were applied in arriving at a diagnosis. It is then not surprising, that different investigators have found different prevalence rates. Furthermore, since inattention, impulsiveness and hyperactivity tend to change with maturity, different prevalence rates are obtained if one investigator includes in his study only children in kindergarten to grade four and other investigators include children in older age groups as well.

Another confounding difficulty in establishing prevalence rates is that many more boys are reported to suffer from this disorder than girls. If all children are pooled together, a different rate is obtained than when only boys are studied. For example, a study conducted in Italy reported that 20% of the boys and only 3% of the girls were affected. However, the combined rate for all children, when boys and girls were pooled, was 12%.

Many prevalence studies use standardized questionnaires by which parents or teachers rate certain behaviors in children. Some questionnaires require the parent or teacher to respond whether a particular symptom such as inattention is present *"sometimes, often or always."* Other questionnaires require the parents or teacher to respond whether the child displays a particular symptom *"not at all, a little, pretty much or very much."* Thus, using different techniques to establish the prevalence of this disorder will produce different results. Nonetheless, when similar techniques are used, there seems to be a general consensus among different studies reported from different countries. About 2 to 3 percent of the girls and 6 to 9 percent of the boys are reported to be affected in studies conducted in the United States, Great Britain, Australia, Germany and China. Somewhat higher prevalence rates are reported from Italy, Spain and New Zealand.

We know now that ADHD is a life-long disorder. Approximately 80% of ADHD children continue experiencing academic and social difficulties in adolescence and in approximately 60% of affected individuals some of their problems linger into adulthood, albeit in altered forms. For example, overt hyperactivity is replaced by more internal restlessness.

It is apparent that ADHD is a relatively common problem that requires our understanding. The question is how to diagnose and differentiate it from similar behaviour disorders that require different approaches to their treatment. This will be discussed in chapter 5.

4   The Causes of ADHD

There are in fact two things, science and opinion; the former begets knowledge, the latter ignorance.

Hippocrates, 460? -377? BC

Until about a dozen years ago we did not know what caused ADHD. There were many theories that still have their advocates. These will be mentioned after a brief discussion of the recent scientific discoveries that have significantly advanced our understanding of the causes of this disorder. We will confine our discussions here to ADHD as a neurological disorder, which, as mentioned previously, is referred to as primary ADHD by some authorities as opposed to other types of inattention caused by chaotic family circumstances, mental health problems in the family or other stress-producing events or situations.

ADHD may be caused by either genetic or environmental factors. In many individuals ADHD is caused by an interaction of genetic and environmental influences.

Genetic Influences

Genetic influences have long been suspected of being the cause of most cases of ADHD based on the following observations:

1. The parents of ADHD children often report that they have experienced similar problems as their affected children. Some of them report they continue suffering from restlessness, inattention and daydreaming.

2. There is an increase in the reported cases of ADHD among the full siblings of ADHD children as compared to their half siblings. On the whole, about 25% of the close relatives of ADHD children also have ADHD whereas only about 5% of the general childhood population has this condition.

3. Many more boys than girls are affected by ADHD suggesting a genetic predisposition in boys. This, however, may be due to a different manifestation of ADHD in girls. Girls with ADHD are often less aggressive physically and exhibit less hyperactivity. They are thus less likely to be referred for evaluation.

4. Studies on the occurrence of ADHD in twins have demonstrated that when one of the twins has ADHD, the likelihood of ADHD in the other twin is much greater if the twins are identical (monozygotic) than if they are non-identical (dizygotic).

These observations have now been supported by recent discoveries of genes involved in the function of the dopamine system within the brain. Dopamine is one of the many neurotransmitters (chemicals manufactured by the brain) that carry the nervous signals amongst brain cells. There is clinical and research findings pointing to an underproduction or a functional impairment of the dopamine system in ADHD individuals which interferes with communication between parts of the brain that regulate attention, planning, impulse control and motor activity. Another important neurotransmitter is norepinephrine, which, among other functions, enhances the inhibitory and executive functions of the brain. These functions will be briefly described at the end of this chapter.

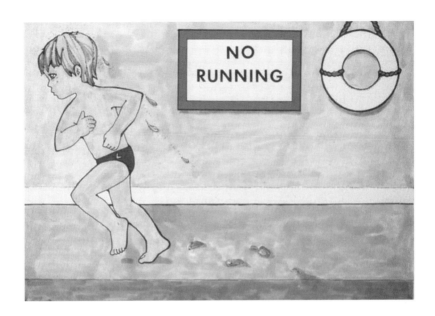

Sophisticated imaging studies have also demonstrated that certain parts of the brain of persons with ADHD are smaller than the identical parts in normal population.

Environmental Factors

Alcohol, Tobacco and Illicit Drugs

Environmental factors include prenatal damage to the growing fetal brain resulting from the mother's excessive alcohol consumption, smoking tobacco and substance abuse. We know that heavy alcohol consumption during pregnancy can lead to the development of fetal alcohol syndrome. This syndrome consists of variable degrees of mental retardation, moderate growth deficiency, abnormal facial structures, a number of other abnormalities, as well as weak attention and hyperactivity. We also know that babies born to smoking mothers are, on the whole, smaller than babies born to non-smokers.

We do not know the possible subtle effects of minimal to moderate alcohol consumption or smoking on the developing fetus. As long as this is not known, it is prudent for pregnant women to refrain from smoking or drinking alcoholic beverages. The same can be said about pregnancy and substance abuse. Since illicit drugs are indulged for their effects on the abusers' brain, it is evident that any substance abuse during pregnancy will have deleterious effect on the developing brain of the fetus.

Poisoning

Environmental poisons such as lead and other toxic metals as well as PCBs (polychlorinated biphenyls) have been implicated, but not proven, to cause ADHD symptoms. It has been suggested that chronic exposures to these toxic agents at concentrations too low to produce the usual clinical signs of poisoning may lead to subtle biochemical changes within the brain and to subsequent development of ADHD symptoms in some children. Up to the present time, we have no definitive evidence of such subtle poisonings.

Nutritional Factors

Essential fatty acids omega 3 (alpha-linolenic acid) and omega 6 (linoleic acid) found naturally in many seeds, seed oils, fish oil (e.g., salmon and tuna) and other foods play an important role in human health. A deficiency of these fatty acids and their derivatives (long chain polyunsaturated fatty acids) adversely affect the development and functions of many organs including the brain. There are a number of reports indicating that a supplement of these fatty acids may improve the reading and spelling skills as well as the behaviour of *some* ADHD children. These reports support the notion of interaction of genetic and environmental factors in the genesis of some cases of ADHD. In some genetically predisposed children, a deficiency or an abnormal metabolism of these fatty acids may lead to the manifestations of learning problems and ADHD behaviors. It appears that such individuals require higher amounts of these fatty acids to function normally.

Zinc plays an important role in the metabolism of essential fatty acids, brain development and many metabolic processes in the brain. Some studies have reported an improvement in the symptoms of ADHD with zinc supplementation. Other mineral such as magnesium, copper, chromium, iron, selenium and calcium and, of course, all vitamins, play significant roles in human metabolism. These minerals and vitamins are collectively referred to as micronutrients as opposed to macronutrients such as proteins, carbohydrates and fats. There are many studies suggesting that supplementing the diet of some sufferers of mood or behaviour disorders (depressed, aggressive, violent) with one or more micronutrients leads to an improvement of their symptoms. It appears that some genetically predisposed people require higher amounts of these micronutrients to function normally. It is quite possible that some ADHD individuals may also fall into this category. There is a need for further studies in this very promising field of relationship between nutritional factors and human behaviour.

Other Suggested Causes of ADHD

Premature Birth

In reviewing the medical history of ADHD children, one often finds that premature birth is more common among them as compared to general childhood population. Since only a segment of prematurely born babies develop ADHD, it can be assumed that premature birth, per se, is not a direct cause of ADHD. Rather, in some prematurely born babies there are developmental deficiencies of certain areas of their brain, areas that regulate attention, freedom from distraction and impulse control.

Maturational Lag

Since the behaviour of ADHD children is abnormal relative to their own age, but resembles those of younger children, it has been suggested that ADHD children are slow in the development of certain functions of their brains. The problem with this assumption is that a lag suggests that eventually these children will "catch up." Unfortunately some of the abnormal behaviors of a significant number of ADHD children persist, although to a lesser degree of severity, into adulthood. Another problem with the notion of a maturational lag is that it encourages some parents or professionals to postpone effective treatments, hoping that the child's brain will eventually mature. During the intervening time, however, the child and his family continue to suffer needlessly.

Brain Injury

Brain injury resulting from severe trauma or infections can cause behavioral changes consistent with the diagnosis of ADHD. However, in the majority of cases of ADHD there is no history of such events. Minor head trauma is very common in childhood and it is difficult to relate them to the development of ADHD. A careful history usually reveals that the child had some or all of the behavioral problems prior to the minor head trauma. In fact, it is likely that the impulsive behaviour of the hyperactive child may have led to his head trauma. Repeated and careful neurological examinations of ADHD children very seldom reveal signs of significant neurological abnormalities. The so-called minor or soft neurological signs, such as poor gross or fine motor coordination skills that are often seen in ADHD children, are difficult to interpret since the same signs are also seen in so many normal, non-ADHD children.

Hormone Abnormalities

Hyperthyroidism or over-activity of the thyroid gland can cause hyperactivity, weak attention and a reduced learning rate. However, this condition also has many other prominent signs and symptoms that make it easily recognizable by the examining physician. It is not necessary to do routine thyroid testing on a child with ADHD.

Sensitivity to Fluorescent Light

Fluorescent light has been suggested by some people as a possible cause of ADHD symptoms in some individuals. Carefully designed experiments have demonstrated conclusively that this is not true.

Food Sensitivity

The relation between food and ADHD is discussed in chapter 10.

Despite the recent scientific findings that leave no doubt that ADHD is a neurological disorder, there are still a few individuals, including some celebrities with no background in science, who believe that ADHD is a behaviour problem with its cause rooted in the child's psychosocial environment. They argue that physicians, in collusion with drug companies and some teachers, have "medicalized" this condition. There is no question that a chaotic home environment, marital discord, mental illness in the family and many other stress-producing situations can lead to behaviour problems in children. Neither is there any doubt that overcrowded classrooms, staffed by inadequately trained teachers, or boredom in a bright child, as well as many other psychosocial factors, can also lead to inattention and other behavioral problems in some children. We also know that an extremely hyperactive child can create chaos both at home and in school, bring out the worst in the family and interfere with the teaching effectiveness of even the most capable teacher. From these observations, however, one can not generalize that the root of all behaviour problems in children is in their psychosocial environments. What can be stated with certainty is that the child's psychosocial environment can influence the severity of ADHD, and especially the degree of impairment and suffering the child may experience.

The classification of the causes of ADHD has obvious therapeutic implications. Clearly, medication will be of no value for a child whose inattention is caused by his family's marital discord or other stress producing situations. On the other hand, medications, particularly stimulant drugs, have a major role in the treatment of ADHD. This will be further discussed in chapter 6, "Management of ADHD." At this juncture, it should only be mentioned that there is some laboratory and clinical evidence that dopamine "deficiency" (impaired production, metabolism, transport or uptake by the receptor sites of dopamine) leads to an under-arousal of certain areas of the brain. This under-arousal makes it difficult for the ADHD individual to resist distraction and to focus attention selectively on those stimuli most important for the task at hand.

This selective attention is the mental process that allows us to recognize and choose the central and most important stimulus from a complex and ever-changing array of individual pieces of information arriving at our brain on a moment-by-moment basis. This ability seems to be dependent upon the availability of appropriate concentration of dopamine within certain areas of our brain. Stimulant drugs increase the concentration or availability of dopamine within these areas, in turn enhancing the ability to focus attention selectively and resist distraction. In this respect, stimulant drugs do not evoke a contradictory (paradoxical) response in ADHD children as was thought to be the case by some in the past (Why give stimulant drugs to hyperactive children?).

It is interesting to note that Dr. Charles C. Bradley, the originator of stimulant therapy in 1937, came to the same conclusion. He suggested that since certain parts of the brain have an inhibitory function over stimuli received by the brain through the peripheral nervous system, any stimulation of these parts would enhance their inhibitory function.

The following may help to explain the inhibitory function of our brains. At all times, the brain receives, continuously and simultaneously, multiple stimuli through our senses. We hear sounds, see objects, smell odors and feel our clothing at the same time. Our brains, however, are programmed to *inhibit* and ignore irrelevant stimuli and concentrate on the most important stimulus. For example, while reading these lines, we may also hear people talk and feel the chair we are sitting on. Subconsciously, however, we ignore everything except the visual stimulus, the written words. This inhibition of irrelevant stimuli is an important part of our brain function. Without it, we would be distracted by every sound, sight and smell, unable to concentrate on what we intend to do. Dr. Bradley suggested that this inhibitory function is impaired in hyperactive children and is restored by Benzedrine. We know now that Benzedrine works primarily on the norepinephrine system which increases the inhibitory and the executive functions of the brain; i.e., our ability to plan, anticipate, initiate, self-monitor and carry out a task to its intended end without being distracted by irrelevant stimuli.

Reason is immortal, all else is mortal.

Pythagoras, circa 582-500 BC

The optimal diagnostic evaluation of ADHD would require the input of a team of professionals consisting of a specially trained physician, the child's teacher, or special education teacher, a psychologist, a social worker and, in some cases, other professionals. Such teams are normally available only in major centres and can handle only a small fraction of children affected by ADHD. In the majority of cases, parents must rely on their family physician or pediatrician to make a diagnosis in consultation with the child's teacher.

Due to the fact that physicians have no precise way of measuring inattention, impulsiveness and hyperactivity, the diagnosis of ADHD remains a relatively difficult task for them. Purposeless over-activity is particularly difficult to measure objectively. A certain amount of activity may be quite normal for a three-year-old child. However, the same amount of activity is regarded as excessive for an eight-year-old. There are no standardized norms of activity, similar to those for height and weight, against which one can measure the child's activity level. A cynic once defined hyperactivity as "the amount of activity that annoys the observer!" Although there are some objective tests available to measure impulsiveness and inattention, complications remain with the definition of these terms.

The difficulties associated with this lack of precise definition have hampered studies of ADHD for a considerable time. Researchers did not have a uniform and precise system of including children in, or excluding them from, their studies. The diagnostic criteria introduced by the American Psychiatric Association, in 1981 and revised in 1987, 1994 and 2000, provided scientists with an additional tool to help them with clinical diagnosis of ADHD.

Diagnostic Criteria for Attention Deficit/Hyperactivity Disorder

(from the *Diagnostic and Statistical Manual* [DSM IV-TR] American Psychiatric Association)

A.   Either (1) or (2):

1.   **inattention**: six (or more) of the following symptoms of inattention have persisted for at least six months to a degree that is maladaptive and inconsistent with developmental level:

a) Often fails to give close attention to details and makes careless mistakes in schoolwork, work, or other activities.

b) Often has difficulty sustaining attention in tasks or play activities.

c) Often does not seem to listen when spoken to directly.

d) Often does not follow through on instructions and fails to finish schoolwork, chores, or duties in the workplace (not due to oppositional behaviour or failure to understand instructions).

e) Often has difficulty organizing tasks and activities.

f) Often avoids, dislikes, or is reluctant to engage in tasks that require sustained mental efforts (such as schoolwork or homework).

g) Often loses things necessary for tasks or activities (e.g., toys, school assignments, pencils, books, or tools).

h) Is often easily distracted by extraneous stimuli.

i) Is often forgetful in daily activities.

2. **Hyperactivity-impulsivity**: six (or more) of the following symptoms of hyperactivity-impulsivity have persisted for at least six months to a degree that is maladaptive and inconsistent with developmental level:

Hyperactivity

a) Often fidgets with hands or feet or squirms in seat.

b) Often leaves seat in classroom or in other situations in which remaining seated is expected.

c) Often runs about or climbs excessively in situations in which it is inappropriate (in adolescents or adults, may be limited to subjective feelings of restlessness).

d) Often has difficulty playing or engaging in leisure activities quietly.

e) Is often "on the go" or often acts as if driven by a motor.

f) Often talks excessively.

Impulsivity

g) Often blurts out answers before questions have been completed.

h) Often has difficulty awaiting turn.

i) Often interrupts or intrudes on others (e.g., butts into conversations or games).

B.   Some hyperactive-impulsive or inattentive symptoms that caused impairment were present before age 7 years.

C.   Some impairment from the symptoms is present in two or more settings (e.g., at school or work or at home).

D.   There must be clear evidence of clinically significant impairment in social, academic, or occupational functioning.

E.   The symptoms do not occur exclusively during the course of a Pervasive Developmental Disorder, or Schizophrenia, or other Psychotic Disorders and are not better accounted for by another mental disorder (e.g., Mood Disorder, Anxiety Disorder, Dissociative Disorders, or a Personality Disorder).

If both Criteria A1 and A2 are met for the past six months DSM IV-TR classifies the diagnosis as ADHD Combined Type.

If criterion A1 is met but criterion A2 is not met for the past six months, DSM IV-TR classifies the diagnosis as ADHD Predominantly Inattentive Type.

If criterion A2 is met but criterion A1 is not met for the past six months, DSM IV-TR classifies the diagnosis as ADHD Predominantly Hyperactive-Impulsive Type.

ADHD can further be classified as *simple or complex.* The simple ADHD refers to individuals who have one of the above subtypes with no other concurrent conditions. Only one in five cases of ADHD can be classified as *simple ADHD.* Four out of five cases are associated with other problems such as learning disabilities, mental retardation, mood disorders, anxiety disorders, etc. These are classified as *complex ADHD.*

As can be seen from the diagnostic criteria there is still a great deal of impreciseness in the definitions. For example: How often is "often"? More often than expected for the child's age?

What is expected of a child of any age depends on the observer's own level of tolerance. There are no precisely defined standards. Unfortunately there are no diagnostic laboratory tests, such as blood or urine tests or X-rays, that are available for many physical disorders. *A careful history taken from the child's caregivers, i.e., parents and teachers, is the most reliable tool currently available for the diagnosis of ADHD.*

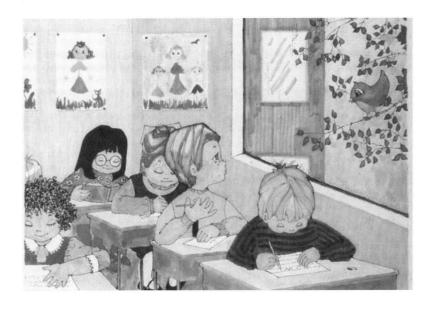

Medical History

Since the behaviour of ADHD children varies from situation to situation (classroom versus physician's office) and from day-to-day in the same situation, it is important for the professionals to observe the child and obtain behavioral reports from his parents and teachers. Inconsistency of behaviour is a characteristic of ADHD children. In the one-on-one situation in the physician's office, ADHD children often behave normally. Their teachers and parents often report completely different behaviour patterns. Experienced professionals rely heavily on these reports, since both teachers and parents have observed the child over a longer period of time and have had the opportunity to compare him with other children of the same age.

There are many standardized parent-teacher questionnaires for the purpose of obtaining information on child behaviour. The best known of these, the *Conners'* parent-teacher questionnaires, are used for identifying ADHD symptoms along with symptoms of possible coexisting problems, such as disruptive behaviour, anxiety disorders, perfectionism and social problems. The information obtained from these behaviour-rating questionnaires is supplemented by the medical history of the child and is used to ascertain whether the child meets the diagnostic criteria developed by the American Psychiatric Association. The abbreviated forms of these questionnaires target only ADHD symptoms and are best suited for the evaluation of a child's response to medication. They are presented on the following pages as examples of the type of questions asked.

Abbreviated Conners' Questionnaires

Parent's Questionnaire

Instructions: Listed below are 14 items concerning children's behaviour or the problems they sometimes have. Read each item carefully and decide how much you think this child has been displaying this behaviour *today*.

Child's Name: _____

Parent's Name: _____

Today's Date: _____

Observation		Frequency			
		Not at all	Just a little	Often	Almost Always
1	Body in constant motion.				
2	Difficulty sitting through a meal.				
3	Constant squirming while watching TV or playing with toys.				
4	Restless in car, church, while shopping, etc.				
5	Keeps changing activities or games.				
6	Starts things without finishing them; does not complete tasks.				
7	Difficulty playing cooperatively with others for more than a few minutes.				
8	Does not seem to listen attentively or hear what you say.				
9	Stares at things for long periods.				
10	Talks too much or too loudly.				
11	Interrupts or interferes with others' conversations or activities.				
12	Mood changes quickly and unpredictably.				
13	Easily frustrated; demands must be immediately.				
14	Acts without thinking.				

Comments:

_____

_____

_____

_____

_____

_____

Teacher's Questionnaire

Instructions: Listed below are 13 items concerning children's behaviour or problems they sometimes have. Read each item carefully and decide how much you think this child has been displaying this behaviour today.

Child's Name: _____

Parent's Name: _____

Today's Date: _____

	Observation	Frequency			
		Not at all	Just a little	Often	Almost Always
1	Difficulty sitting still or excessive fidgeting, restlessness.				
2	Difficulty staying seated, often on the go.				
3	Starts things without finishing them; does not complete tasks.				
4	Doesn't seem to listen attentively when spoken to.				
5	Has difficulty following oral direction.				
6	Easily distracted, difficulty concentrating.				
7	Difficulty staying with a play activity.				
8	Acts before thinking.				
9	Has difficulty organizing work.				
10	Needs a lot of supervision.				
11	Interacts poorly with other children.				
12	Demands must be met immediately easily distracted.				
13	Mood changes quickly, cries, temper outbursts.				

Comments:

_____

_____
_____
_____
_____
_____

There are other comprehensive questionnaires, such as SNAP IV, that provide for an overall assessment of the child's behaviour at home and school and point to possible coexisting problems that may require additional therapeutic interventions. The process of diagnosis is not complete unless the presence or absence of these disorders is ascertained. The medical history should also inquire about the following:

- The onset, severity and frequency of the troublesome behaviors and their possible precipitating factors.

- Any history of mental health problems or childhood ADHD in the parents and their siblings as well as the child's siblings.

- The number of the siblings in the family and the amount and severity of sibling rivalry.

- The presence of marital discord and other family stressors.

- How the family is coping with the ADHD child and what supports are available to them in the community.

- The type and consistency of parental disciplinary measures and the child's response to them.

- Maternal health problems during pregnancy and the events associated with labor, delivery and the early days of the child's life.

- Feeding problems in the child during infancy and sleep problems that the child may have.
- Medications that the child may be taking.

Commonly Reported Behaviour Patterns

The behaviour of ADHD children changes with age and maturity. Furthermore, they do not always exhibit the full range of abnormal behaviour that could possibly occur at their age. Appropriate treatment may modify their behaviour in a helpful way. The following is a brief presentation of commonly *reported* behaviour problems of ADHD children. It should be mentioned, however, that carefully designed studies have demonstrated that some of these reported behaviors do not, in fact, occur more frequently in ADHD children than they do in the normal childhood population.

Infancy

Hyperactivity and irritability may be noticeable features during the first year of life. The baby may be constantly wiggling and difficult to hold. Some mothers report excessive motor activity even before the child is born. In this stage of the child's development, his hyperactivity is not usually bothersome to his parents. They are more troubled by his poor patterns of feeding and sleeping.

The child is usually a poor feeder and is colicky. In most infants, the colic disappears during the first few months of life. In children who are subsequently recognized as ADHD, the colic may be present throughout the entire first year of life. During this time, the child may demand almost constant attention by fussing and crying. He may seem to need continuous entertainment. He may also have a difficult time falling asleep and may frequently wake up during the night. This may continue long beyond the age when most infants begin to sleep through the night. After the infant learns to crawl or walk, his hyperactivity and curiosity may make him a first-class explorer. This usually leads to more than his share of accidents through such activities as climbing up and falling from furniture, and crawling under the kitchen sink to help himself to detergents, solvents, bleach or whatever else he can find. He may seem to have several busy hands and is usually several steps ahead of his parents. Of course, at this age, no one expects a baby to be entirely focused and restrained. A great deal of acting without thinking is quite normal in infancy. What sets these children apart is their unusual difficulty to learn from past experience, which includes their parents' efforts to shape their behaviour.

Preschool Years

During the preschool years, the excessive motor activity persists and may become even more prominent. Difficulties with attention and impulse control become more evident now. The child seems to go from activity to activity, and unless his parents or his play school teacher stand next to him, he will not remain with any activity for more than a few short periods of time. He grabs toys from other children, disrupting their play and showing aggression toward them. He manages to become very unpopular with other children since he always wants to have his own way. He can learn the rules of good behaviour, but somehow he seems to be unable to follow these rules unless he is constantly reminded. Punishment of any sort does not seem to have lasting effect on him. His impulsiveness continues, as does his tendency to be accident-prone. He may dash across the street without looking or get himself fearlessly into dangerous situations. Sleep difficulties may continue. He may wake up in the middle of the night to raid the refrigerator, turn the television on or otherwise explore the household, wondering why everyone else is asleep. Some ADHD children are also early risers and often are not in a happy mood when they wake up.Mood swings and temper tantrums may become apparent at this age.

Early School Years

The most troublesome problem for the child in his early school years is poor ability to attend to learning tasks. About 20 to 30 percent of ADHD children also have various degrees of learning disability. Even if they have the ability to learn, they cannot attend long enough to do so. The ADHD child starts a task but leaves it incomplete because he is distracted by everything around him. Consequently he falls behind in his schoolwork. If he is bright, however, and has no associated learning disability, he may learn quite well in spite of his inattentiveness. He may not walk excessively around the classroom but he fidgets and squirms constantly. He talks loudly and out of turn and generally disrupts the classroom activities. He tends to answer the questions before the teacher has finished a sentence, that is, if he is not daydreaming. His teacher reports that often he seems to be in a different world. He is disorganized and his work is quite messy. His disregard for the rules continues, and thus, he is often left out of organized games. He may feel rejected and lonely and his self-esteem begins to suffer. His disturbed sleep pattern may continue and he may now have nightmares or other signs of distress. His parents may become aware of snoring and or sleep apnea. His mood swings may also continue and his low tolerance for frustration will lead to impatience, increased temper outbursts and aggression toward his peers, teacher and parents.

Adolescence

Around 10 or 11 years, the ADHD child shows a noticeable decrease in hyperactivity but may still be fidgety and restless. During this period his poor impulse control severely interferes with his social relationships. His effort at socialization may be awkward or insensitive to others' feelings. He may be craving friendship but becomes more isolated and, in frustration, he may engage in antisocial behaviour. He is more likely than his peers to experiment with illicit drugs. His social and academic failure may lead to further isolation and depression. Inattention and impulsiveness may continue into adulthood. In a young adult, hyperactivity is replaced by restlessness. Underachievement, social awkwardness and frustrations may become   ongoing problems.

ADHD in adolescents will be further discussed in chapter 12.

Medical Examination

Children of school age are often brought to a physician at the request of their teachers. Not infrequently, the parents report that the child's teacher has recommended a medical examination for the child, including tests such as an EEG (brain wave recordings). Occasionally, the parents ask for a brain scan or other expensive investigations.

It is the experience of all physicians who have worked with ADHD and learning-disabled children that medical examinations and routine blood and urine tests in these children almost invariably produce normal results. Likewise, detailed neurological examination of these children usually reveals no significant findings of concern. Of course, this does not mean that a medical examination is useless or unwarranted. The experienced physician knows that a thorough medical examination, including an assessment of the child's hearing and vision, is essential to rule out any possible physical problems and assures the parents of thoroughness of investigation. It also increases the parents' confidence in their physician and adherence to recommended treatment options.

Frequently one finds ADHD children who show some signs of delay in the maturation of their nervous system. They may have poor ability to balance on one foot, hop on one foot, or turn their palms face up and face down rapidly. They may also have difficulty knowing the right and left sides of their own body. These so-called soft neurological signs are, however, also seen in many children with no attention or learning problems. Minor changes in electroencephalograms are also seen in many ADHD as well as in non-ADHD children. Routine EEGs are of no value in the diagnosis of ADHD but are most useful if there is any suggestion from the history that the child may have a seizure problem. Promising new developments in the measurements of brain activity through quantitative analysis of encephalograms are available now, as are brain scans measuring brain functions. Although these expensive techniques may enable us to differentiate between learning and behaviour disorders originating from brain malfunction and those of environmental origin, they are presently investigative tools and have no role in the routine diagnosis of ADHD.

Some investigators have reported subtle differences between the brainwaves of ADHD children and those of typical, non-ADHD children. These investigators claim success in normalizing the symptoms of ADHD through modifying the brainwaves using biofeedback. This potentially useful treatment tool is presently in experimental stage and not generally available. Some investigators also question their cost/benefit efficiency.

All told, there is no specific or definitive medical, neurological or laboratory tests that can be used for making a reliable diagnosis of ADHD. There is no better substitute to a thorough medical history obtained from the parents and teachers.

Psychological Tests (S. Maunula)

While there is no definitive medical or psychological test for ADHD, psychological assessment can be very helpful in suggesting and confirming diagnosis. Psychological tests can also identify learning difficulties and emotional problems which may be associated with ADHD. Of course, psychological test results always need to be understood in context of the developmental history of the child and his current situation.

The most commonly used tests of intelligence have been the Wechsler scales, of which the Wechsler Intelligence Scale for Children – Fourth Edition (WISC-IV) is the most recent version (2003). Both Canadian and American children have been tested on the WISC-IV, so that a child's mental abilities may be compared to his own age group and nationality. Alternatively, the Stanford-Binet Intelligence Scale (fifth edition in 2003), the Woodcock-Johnson Tests of Cognitive Ability (third version in 2001), or other intelligence tests may be used by some psychologists. While the WISC-IV provides a measure of general intelligence, it also considers different ways that a child understands information. The WISC-IV provides scales of both verbal comprehension and nonverbal reasoning. Furthermore, it measures auditory memory and visual processing speed. Certain subtests of the WISC-IV can be reflective of the attention and motivation of the child. While there is no typical ADHD pattern of strengths and weaknesses found on the WISC-IV (or other intelligence measures), children's concentration and persistence for various tasks may be observed during testing.

Children with ADHD have general ability levels which cover the full range of intelligence found within the general population. However, there can sometimes be large differences among the various cognitive "factors" which lead us to suspect learning problems. Verbal abilities may be much stronger than non-verbal reasoning, suggesting learning difficulties relating to poor visual perception. Conversely, strong visual perception and weak verbal abilities may suggest a language-based learning problem. Extremely low or borderline intellectual functioning is sometimes found among children with attention problems, as these students have much difficulty keeping up with a regular school curriculum. Conversely, some students with ADHD may be identified as "gifted," given superior performance on these tests.

Behaviour rating scales, completed by the child's parents and teacher(s), are extremely useful in determining whether a child's attention and behaviour represent significant problems both at home and in the classroom. Earlier in this chapter we mentioned the Conners' parent/teacher behaviour rating scales and presented their abbreviated forms. Another behaviour rating scale is SNAP-IV (Swanson, Nolan and Pelham, 1983). These scales are specific to ADHD and other disruptive behaviours, and are most useful in targeting inattentive and hyperactive-impulsive symptoms. They are not only helpful in confirming the diagnosis of ADHD but also in measuring a child's response to treatment. There are other broad rating scales, such as the ASEBA (Achenbach System of Empirically–Based Assessment, 2001), Child Behaviour Checklist and Teacher Rating Form, or the Behaviour Assessment System for Children (BASC-second edition, 2004). These scales are helpful in identifying which clusters of emotions and behaviors are of "clinical" concern. That is to say, are some characteristics of the child with ADHD more extreme than observed in the general childhood population?

A relatively new instrument, called the Behaviour Rating Inventory of Executive Function (BRIEF) is starting to be used to evaluate "*executive functions*" of children in their home and school environments. The term, executive function, represents a collection of interrelated functions of the brain that is responsible for goal-oriented, problem-solving behaviour. It includes planning, initiating, anticipating, self-monitoring, judgement and completing a task to its intended end without being distracted. Although not specifically for use with ADHD children, this parent or teacher questionnaire helps to identify difficulties with the child's "high level" cognitive functioning, such as impulse control, "shifting activities," emotional control, initiative, organizational skills, self monitoring and working memory. (Working memory is the capacity of the brain to hold information actively "online" in the service of problem-solving. It is an integral aspect of executive function. It is also referred to as short-term memory.) It is important to consider these functions when planning a school program for the child or one for helping him do his homework and other daily activities.

For older children, there are self-report versions of the ASEBA and BASC-2 forms. Dr. Thomas Brown has also developed self-report scales of ADD for adolescents and adults.

Some computerized tests of vigilance, such as the Continuous Performance Test (CPT), have been used to differentiate children with ADHD from those with no attention problems. However, these tests have sometimes mistakenly identified children as having ADHD without other collaborating evidence. Also, some children with ADHD enjoy the fast pace and novelty of the computerized test and respond well initially but then get bored with it when testing continues or is repeated. Based on these weaknesses, the CPT is not recommended as a single measure for the diagnosis of ADHD.

Tests of academic achievement are also used to determine the student's level of reading, mathematics, spelling and written expression. A psychologist, resource teacher or education consultant may give a broad test of academic skills and/or diagnostic tests in specific subject areas. The Wechsler Individual Achievement Test (second edition, 2002), Woodcock-Johnson Tests of Achievement or Kaufman Tests of Educational Achievement are commonly used broad measures. If a child's achievement in one or more subject areas is substantially below his or her level of intelligence, then a learning disability may be identified.

Allergy Tests

Some parents ask for allergy tests for their children, believing that allergies play a role in ADHD. No one has ever demonstrated a convincing cause-and-effect relationship between allergy and ADHD, similar to those between pollens and hayfever or peanuts and hives. There is some evidence that immunological disorders (including allergies) are seen more often in ADHD and learning disabled children than in the typical childhood population. The relationship between food and ADHD is discussed in chapter 10.

Hair Analysis

Occasionally parents ask for a hair analysis of their children to diagnose potential poisoning with lead or other toxic substances. Many commercial laboratories offer hair analysis services and often give the results of their tests in impressive computer printouts. Unfortunately, commercial hair analysis has not proven to be a reliable test for this purpose. (A sample of hair from a child, divided in two parts, and sent to the same laboratory under two different fictitious names, produced two completely different results for one of this book's authors.) Even if commercial hair analysis were reliable and accurate, its results would not necessarily reflect the status of the tested elements in the child's brain or elsewhere in his body. Better tests for detecting environmental toxins in blood and urine are available and can be ordered by the child's physician if indicated on the basis of the child's history and medical examination. The indication for such tests in ADHD children is extremely uncommon.

In summary, the diagnosis of ADHD requires a careful attention to the child's history obtained by interviewing his parents and, whenever possible, the child himself. This information, together with behaviour rating questionnaires completed by parents and teachers, medical examination, as well as psychological and educational tests are sufficient for a reasonably accurate diagnosis of ADHD.

6   Management of ADHD: Drug Therapy

Thiru Govender, MD

Healing is a matter of time, but it is also sometimes a matter of opportunity.

Hippocrates, 460 ?–377 ? BC

The optimal treatment of ADHD is a combination of various approaches; i.e., behaviour therapy (including, when needed, psychotherapy), medications, family therapy, social skills training, parenting skills training, classroom management and family support groups.

As an integral part of a multimodal and multidisciplinary approach in treating children with ADHD, medications have an important role in its overall management. They have been used now for more than several decades and have been well investigated. To date, there are over 10 000 studies on ADHD and its management published in respected medical and psychological journals attesting to their safety and efficacy as well as addressing their possible side effects. At this early point in the chapter, it must be re-emphasized that medications are most effective when used in conjunction with a comprehensive behavioral, social and academic management program, designed to meet the needs of each individual with ADHD. When used as a part of such programs, they can be very helpful in improving a student's academic function and socialization with their peers in the classroom and outside of it.

Before a decision is made to use medications it is extremely important to obtain and review information from the parents and the school regarding the child's functional level and degree of severity of symptoms of ADHD. When it is decided that medications may be beneficial to the child, their use, mode of action, expected effects and possible side effects must be discussed with the child's parents, teachers and, if indicated, with the child himself.

It is also extremely important to discuss with the parents, the student and the school that during the initial trial period, while the child is started on a medication, there may be changes made to the dose of the medication depending on the child's response. Indeed, the medication itself may be changed. During this trial period, the prescribing physician should remain in regular contact with the child's parents and teachers to determine the child's response to medication. After it is determined that the child is responding in a positive manner to the medication, it is important for the physician to have periodic contact with the school since the child's teacher is in an excellent position to observe the child's progress and his response to medication.

Mode of Action

The effectiveness of psycho-stimulant medication in treating ADHD was, for many years, an enigma. The question was how a psycho-stimulant medication helped "settle" children who were hyperactive. Over the years it became apparent that the core symptoms of ADHD, i.e., inattention, distractibility, impulsivity and hyperactivity were the results of a weakness at the level of the synaptic junction in certain areas of the brain and associated with a deficiency and altered metabolism of chemicals called neurotransmitters.

A synapse is a junction of two nerves where messages are transferred from a sending nerve to a receiving nerve with the help of chemical compounds called neurotransmitters. There are a number of neurotransmitters that are associated with ADHD, primarily dopamine and noradrenalin (also known as norepinephrine). Focused attention is a function of the prefrontal area of the brain and it is in this area where dopamine and noradrenalin neurotransmitters are found to be deficient.

Both the psycho-stimulant and non-stimulant medications work by increasing the efficacy of the neurotransmitters and thus improve focused attention and reduce distractibility and impulsivity.

There is much research continuing to further help us understand how these neurotransmitters affect our ability to pay attention and how the medications work at that level.

Myths and Controversies

Over the years a number of myths and controversies surrounding the use of medication in the treatment of ADHD have emerged.

Over-prescription

There has been much discussion regarding physicians over-prescribing stimulants for ADHD. While this may have been true to some extent in the past, based on the studies conducted in the United States, there is minimal to no evidence of over-prescription of the stimulant medications at the present time. There has been an increase in the use of stimulant medications for the treatment of ADHD and for longer periods of time, which indicates a greater recognition of this condition as a neurological disorder and the efficacy of its treatment.

Addiction

There are also concerns that psycho-stimulant medications used for the treatment of ADHD are addictive and lead to the use of other banned substances. This has not been found to be the case in many published studies. In fact, long-term and consistent treatment with psycho-stimulants has been shown to protect against substance abuse. It is also important to note that studies have also shown that untreated ADHD in children can lead to substance abuse in adulthood.

Interference with Growth

Another concern is that psycho-stimulants may interfere with the action of growth hormone and stunt growth. In this area, there have been a number of studies completed and about one half of them show there is a statistically significant decrease in height growth velocity and the other half show no significant decrease in height growth velocity. Similar concerns have been expressed regarding the appetite suppressing effects of psycho-stimulant medications on height growth. There are no definite studies to confirm these concerns. Research in these important areas continues. If there is any delay in the height growth, discontinuation of the medication usually leads to a catch up and normalization of the height. When a child is on psycho-stimulant medications, his height is plotted on a regular basis to ensure that his height growth velocity remains at the appropriate and normal rate. Linear height growth of 3 to 5 cm in one year is considered a normal growth velocity, indicating normal growth hormone production.

Tic Disorders

Another concern is that stimulants may cause tics and complex tic disorders such as Tourette's syndrome. It is known that latent (inactive) tics can become apparent when children take psycho-stimulant medications. Psycho-stimulant medications, however, do not cause the tic disorder. They may unmask the genetic potential for that child to have this condition. In other words, for those individuals who have the genetic potential to have a tic disorder, the medication may bring about the symptoms sooner than if they were not on medication. Interestingly, if children do have tic disorders prior to treatment with psycho-stimulant medications, a number of them will actually lose their tics after treatment with these medications. Obviously this is another area that will require ongoing research.

Concerns About Efficacy

Finally it has been stated that psycho-stimulant medications do not really help ADHD. Psycho-stimulant medications work very effectively in the *majority* of ADHD cases. There have been many well-conducted studies confirming the efficacy of psycho-stimulant medication in treating ADHD. The noted improvements in academic performance, in socialization skills and in family relationships are the best indicators of the efficacy of psycho-stimulants. It is important to know that ADHD is a highly prevalent, persistent and impairing brain disorder and one that is significantly improved by a combination of behavioral management strategies and the use of medications.

Medications in Use in Canada

The short acting or immediate release psycho-stimulants were the first medications used in treating ADHD. **Ritalin** (methylphenidate) and **Dexedrine** (dextroamphetamine) were used for a number of years prior to the introduction of the longer acting medications.

A disadvantage of Ritalin and Dexedrine is that they are short acting medications, usually reaching a peak concentration in the bloodstream two or three hours after ingestion and are excreted after three to four hours. Therefore, the clinical effect is short lived and requires dosing two or three times a day, a frequency that is not acceptable to many students in school. Also side effects such as irritability (rebound hyperactivity) are common.

Ritalin SR (sustained release) has a longer duration of action of about six to eight hours but side effects are similar to short acting Ritalin. Nonetheless, Ritalin SR was used for a number of years.

Dexedrine spansules also have approximately an eight hour duration of action. They are taken once a day, in most cases in the morning, but also have side effects such as appetite suppression, which is mostly noticeable at lunchtime. It would appear that with the Dexedrine spansules there is less rebound hyperactivity compared to the other medications. Dexedrine spansules are still prescribed by many physicians.

Although these medications work extremely well, their limited duration of action was a major disadvantage. Many parents were noting that their children were doing extremely well in school but experienced difficulties in after school extracurricular activities. Or, after coming home they were experiencing difficulties in socializing with their friends in the neighborhood. They also had significant problems doing homework. As a result, a consensus developed that a medication that worked for approximately 12 to 14 hours would be ideal. This would help the ADHD children during their school hours and continue to help them with their extra-curricular activities, socialization and completion of homework.

Thus newer forms of long acting methylphenidate (Concerta) and dextroamphetamine (Adderall XR) were developed with a duration of action of about 12 to 14 hours.

Concerta looks like a tablet. However, under the digestible outer coating of the tablet, there is a capsule which has three compartments, two of which contain the active medication and one has "a push chamber." The medication is slowly pushed through a laser-drilled hole in the capsule providing the 12-hour effect.

Adderall XR is also a capsule containing a number of tiny medication beads that are released in a slow fashion over a 12-hour period.

Adderall XR was recalled in February 2005 due to cardiac effects noted in some children and adults. Health Canada withdrew the medication whilst in the USA the medication was not withdrawn. After further research by Health Canada, Adderall XR was re-released for the treatment of ADHD in September 2005.

A non-stimulant medication called **atomoxetine (Strattera)** was developed and shown to have the same effect on the neurotransmitters at the synaptic junction. Being a non-stimulant medication, it was felt that the commonly noted side effects seen with psycho-stimulants, such as appetite suppression and insomnia, would be less pronounced. This would appear to be the case. There are, however, a small number of children who still experience a decrease in appetite and decreased sleep while on the Strattera. Strattera also works for a longer period of time, anywhere up to 20 to 24 hours. This is especially important for children who have difficulty with morning routines due to their ADHD. The preschool hours become less stressful for the child and his family. Atomoxetine use in children with ADHD is relatively new in Canada but has been in use in the United States for about three years at the time of this writing.

Other delivery systems such as a skin patch have been developed but are not available in Canada as of mid 2006.

Other medications have been used and continue to be used in conjunction with the above-noted psycho-stimulants and non-stimulants. They include **Imipramine** (a tricyclic anti-depressant), **Clonidine**, and anti-depressants called SSRI's (selective serotonin re-uptake inhibitors) such as **Prozac** and **Zoloft**. These groups of medications are used to treat complex cases of ADHD where there are coexisting conditions such as depression or severe behavioral concerns. As these medications are not commonly used for treating simple ADHD, they will not be further discussed here.

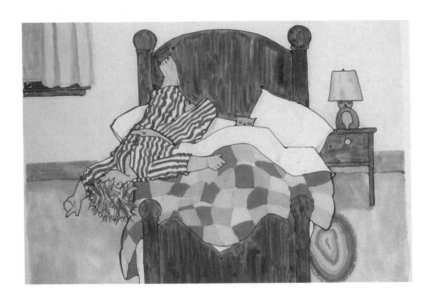

Drug Therapy in Preschool Children

Psycho-stimulant drugs are not commonly used for the management of ADHD in preschool children. Behaviour management remains the main approach to its treatment in this age group. If behaviour management is not sufficient to alleviate the symptoms, medications may be used. However, these preschool children would require more frequent follow up to monitor their response to medications and the potential side effects of drugs. On the whole, the diagnosis and management of the ADHD in preschool children present more difficulties than in older age groups because other behavioral problems in preschool children mimic ADHD. When ADHD is suspected in a preschool child, it is strongly recommended that the child be referred to a multi-disciplinary ADHD clinic, a developmental pediatrician or a child psychiatrist.

Side Effects of Psycho-stimulant Medications

All psycho-stimulant medications described thus far have similar side effects that are often mild and have short duration. When choosing a medication for ADHD, every effort is made to use the dose that is appropriate for the child based on the child's weight and his clinical needs. Side effects appear to be more common with higher doses. With close communication between the physician, parents and teachers ultimately the most appropriate dose for the child can be found, i.e., a dose with greatest effectiveness and the least amount of side effects. The following are the most commonly observed side effects:

Appetite suppression is commonly noted at lunchtime when the medication is at a peak level of concentration in the blood. Various modification of nutrition habits and eating patterns can be used to help children counteract this side effect and to ensure adequate nutrition over the day. For example, a nutritious snack at bedtime to compensate for reduced food intake during the regular meal times can be very effective. Close monitoring of the child's weight, height and growth velocity is important to follow as noted previously.

Insomnia or difficulty falling asleep is another commonly noted side effect. Some ADHD children are quite restless and have difficulty settling to sleep. A small number of children have what is termed a reversal in awake and sleep cycles and these individuals are "night time people" in that they are alert, active and productive late at night but tend to have difficulty staying awake during the day. The longer acting psycho-stimulants seem to settle the restless children and help them sleep better, but do not appear to have effect on the second group of "night time" individuals. Various relaxation techniques may also be employed to help the children sleep better at night.

Abdominal pain and headache. Some children complain of non-specific and vague symptoms of abdominal pain and headaches. It is important for the parents to report to their physician, who by taking a history and completing a physical examination, will determine whether this is a side effect or is related to other medical problems. It is our experience that in the majority of cases, the abdominal pain and the headaches are short lived and tend to disappear on their own while the child is taking the medication.

Rebound hyperactivity. Some children especially those taking the shorter acting forms of the medications, may experience rebound hyperactivity as the medication is wearing off. This irritability or moody behaviour seems to be less prevalent in the longer acting medications. These side effects are also of short duration and seem to be helped in some cases by having a healthy snack and by allowing the child to have a rest or a brief nap.

When a child is on a psycho-stimulant medication, it is important to assess his blood pressure and heart rate on a regular basis. However, elevations in blood pressure and heart rate are not commonly seen in children taking psycho-stimulants. More recently there have been concerns that taking psycho-stimulants and non-stimulants may affect the heart rhythm, which may lead to sudden death and/or stroke. There have been thirty such cases investigated in North America. There is, however, no conclusive evidence that those cases were directly linked to the medication being used. Further studies are showing that the side effects are not more common in children and adults taking psycho-stimulants compared to those who are not taking psycho-stimulants. In other words the incidence of these "side effects" is no greater than it is in the general population. Nonetheless, when prescribing these medications to any child or adult who has a structural defect of the heart or any other rhythm abnormality, the medications should be used with caution and with very close monitoring and after consultation with a cardiologist. In those children and adults who do not have a history of structural heart problems or known rhythm defects, Health Canada has suggested that no further investigations such as EKG's are necessary prior to initiating the medication.

Recently there were some concerns about liver damage when taking the non-stimulant atomoxetine (Strattera). However, there were only two cases, one in a child and one in an adult, reported in over 2 million prescriptions written. Both these individuals had complete reversal to normal of the liver function on cessation of the medication.

Also recently, with Strattera, there have been reports of concerns that there may be increased suicidal ideation while on this medication. Again, all the reports to date have suggested that the incidence of suicidal ideation in children or adults taking Strattera is no more than that in the general population.

An infrequent concern of some parents is that their child has become excessively subdued or depressed. While this can happen, in the majority of cases the parents who have been accustomed to the child's hyperactivity, may interpret his reduced activity level as being abnormal. This is particularly the case when a well-meaning friend, neighbour or relative suggests that the child has become a "zombie." Parents must discuss their concern with their physician before reducing the dose or discontinuing the medication on their own.

There is potential for side effects with any prescribed medication including those prescribed for the treatment of ADHD. One always needs to balance the potential side effects with the positive effects of the medication in the total functioning of the child or adult treated for any medical condition. With regards to ADHD, the non-treatment of the condition may lead to more serious problems in the future.

Psychological side effects of medications used in the treatment of ADHD may be either beneficial or harmful to the child. An enhanced sense of self-esteem resulting from improved academic performance and interpersonal relations is obviously a plus for the child. However, if the medication reinforces the child's belief that he has no control over his own behaviour; that he has to take his pill in order to fight external forces that influence his behaviour, he may develop a distorted view of his personal responsibility for his actions. This undesirable mindset may be reinforced by remarks by the child's teacher, parents, siblings or peers such as, *"did you take your pill today?"* or *"go take your pill,"* whenever he shows a minor deviation in his behaviour. It is the responsibility of the physicians, parents and teachers to emphasize to the child that he is responsible for his own behaviour, and that the pill only helps him in his efforts. In the same vein, any improvement in the child's behaviour and interpersonal relationships should be credited to the child and not to the medication.

One of the beneficial effects of the medication is a change in the parents and teacher's attitude toward the child as a result of his improved behaviour. Studies have shown that parents become less directive and less critical of their children following stimulant therapy. This positive change of attitude in adults toward the child can only be beneficial to the child's emotional well-being in the long run.

Cost. Although not a side effect, a drawback to the longer acting medications is the cost. However, there are many drug plans, both private and public, which will cover the cost of these medications with the appropriate documentation.

Alternative Therapies

Over the years, there have been a number of alternative therapies suggested for the management of ADHD. Unfortunately, good clinical evidence and research have not supported many of these treatment strategies. There are some suggestions that these alternative therapies may have a role in conjunction with the traditional treatment for ADHD. Therefore, it is important for the individuals who are advocating use of these alternative therapies to work in conjunction with researchers to provide the evidence about their efficacy.

Many of these alternative therapies may cause harmful side effects. There is very little regulation as to how some compounds used in alternative therapies are manufactured and what quality control, if any, was in place during the manufacturing process.

The suggestion that many of the alternative therapies are "natural" does not negate the fact that the active components in many of these "natural" and herbal remedies are in fact medications and chemicals. Any medication or chemical that we use for therapeutic purposes should be studied vigorously and presented in well-respected publications prior to recommending their use in children.

The Canadian Pediatric Society, in 2003, issued a position statement on the use of alternative therapies and is recommended as a source of information. See suggested readings and websites.

There are a number of therapies suggested, such as dietary changes, the use of substances that contain multivitamins including essential fatty acids and multiple vitamin supplements. Prior to using any of these, it is strongly recommended that the individuals seek the advice of their pharmacist and physician. The active ingredients of some alternative "natural" remedies may adversely interfere with the medication prescribed by their physician. The relationship between diet and ADHD is further discussed in chapter 10.

Other therapies such as chiropractic therapy, vision therapy, homeopathy, etc., have all been suggested as being beneficial for children and adults with ADHD. There is, however, very little clinical evidence to support these claims. One drug that has been promoted in the past as a natural therapy, namely **Ephedra**, has been associated with fatalities and is condemned by most experts.

To summarize, there may be some benefit in using alternative therapies in conjunction with the traditional treatment of medication and behavioral management strategies. However, good clinical trials are required prior to recommending them.

Adenoidectomy

Children who have obstructive sleep apnea (temporary cessation of breathing during sleep), often associated with snoring, suffer from poor sleep patterns and experience fatigue during awake hours. The fatigue may be associated with behaviour problems, inattention and overall poor school performance. These symptoms are exacerbated in children who have ADHD as well. These children may show some improvement in their behaviour and school performance following adenoidectomy. They must, however, have a thorough pediatric assessment to determine whether a referral to a sleep evaluation centre or for adenoidectomy is required.

7   Behaviour Management

Stephen Maunula, MSc, Psychologist

The sweetest of all sounds is praise.

Xenophon 434?-355? BC

It has been well demonstrated that the most effective treatment for symptoms of ADHD is stimulant medication. Even though inattentive and hyperactive-impulsive symptoms may be minimized in up to 80 percent of children with ADHD through the proper dosage and timing of stimulant medication, there are often disruptive or unproductive behaviors that require further management. Furthermore, behaviour management is the main approach to treating ADHD children under six years of age since psycho-stimulant drugs are not commonly prescribed for this age group.

While children with ADHD are capable of learning new ways of behaving, it is understood that because of their attention problems and impulsive nature, it takes many repeated attempts to teach them a lesson that other children may learn much more quickly. Oftentimes the lesson needs to be taught with enhanced cues to gain their interest and with very clear, direct messages as to what is expected in their behaviour. When a child learns and behaves in a way that is expected of him, he should be rewarded for his efforts in a variety of meaningful ways. It is important that parents and teachers help their children to avoid discouragement from social and academic failure, which often results from untreated ADHD, by teaching them acceptable ways to behave.

Reinforcement

Behaviour management (or behaviour modification) is based on some well-established social learning principles. The main principle is that people will behave in certain ways if they are reinforced (rewarded) for their efforts. Reinforcement refers to any means that increases the likelihood of the recurrence of a desired behaviour. Positive reinforcement may take many different forms. The most immediate social rewards are **attention and praise**. When one closely monitors a child and gives positive attention to his efforts, then that child will likely behave in ways that are pleasing to adults. However, when adults are preoccupied with other things, thereby largely ignoring their child, then he may behave in a disruptive way, which receives negative attention. The task, then, is to pay attention to and reward your child when he is behaving well, rather than give negative attention or punishment only when he is disobedient or behaving in a bothersome way. For some children, gaining attention for disruptive behaviour is better than receiving no attention in busy households or classrooms. If children are ignored for quiet, calm behaviour, and they get a big reaction from adults when they disrupt the smooth flow of activities, then they are more likely to disrupt things again to get some attention, even negative attention, from their parent or teacher.

There are many natural and creative ways of providing positive reinforcement for children. Besides positive attention and praise for a child's efforts, adults, or even peers (classmates and siblings) can provide social and activity rewards to encourage cooperative and productive behaviour. Social recognition can be a powerful motivator. We all like to be acknowledged for our efforts and good deeds. Words of encouragement from parents and teacher, certificates of achievement, and peer nominations can help build self-esteem and confidence in the child, as well as promote good behaviour. Activity rewards, such as playing a video game alone, a board game with a preferred partner, and trips to the science centre, skateboard park, swimming pool or community recreation centre, may be used as "reinforcers" after particularly good days or weeks. When you make time to join your child/student in these activities, you are not only rewarding his good behaviour but are also building positive parent-child or teacher-student relationships.

Some children, especially young ones, are mainly interested in tangible rewards, such as candy, snacks, stickers, toys, trading cards, etc. Children with ADHD, who may not be hungry at regular mealtimes because their appetites are suppressed by stimulant medication, need to be offered nutritious snacks after school or later in the evening when they are hungry. Edible rewards should only be the extra treats that you, as the parent, judge to be reasonable. Remember that something is rewarding only if your child really enjoys it, but you must reserve the right to decide what is reasonable for a family's budget and appropriate for your child.

To address a common misgiving or complaint of parents or teachers, *positive reinforcement is **not** the same thing as bribery*. Positive reinforcement is the principle of delivering a reward after the expected, desirable behaviour has occurred, so as to increase the likelihood that the behaviour will be repeated in the future. Bribery is the offering of an incentive (money or a favor) to someone *before* an expected act is committed, in an attempt to influence his or her conduct. Bribes are often given to coerce people into wrongdoing, not good deeds! While most of us, as adults, continue to work and behave in socially accepted ways without tangible reinforcers, we are occasionally recognized and rewarded for our efforts, which then motivates us to continue our work and pro-social behaviour patterns. There is still the paycheque or the affection of our loved ones that "keeps us going."

A comment about the commonly misunderstood term negative reinforcement: negative reinforcement is not the same thing as negative attention or punishment. Negative reinforcement refers to the strengthening of behaviour when an *adverse stimulus,* like any unpleasant condition, is *withdrawn.* For example, a child may finally clean his room and keep doing so just to end his parent's nagging or yelling. While negative reinforcement may be the reason some children with ADHD eventually comply with requests, it is not a recommended approach to managing behaviour.

The above principles of reinforcement apply when positive (desirable) behaviors can be identified or "targeted" for attainment. Well-meaning adults often focus on negative behaviors and react in dramatic ways after hectic and stressful days. The challenge, then, is to target behaviors that are the positive "flip side" of negative behaviors. For example, at home, if your child is constantly throwing his coat on the floor and tracking mud into the house with his shoes, then the positive target behaviors might be "takes shoes off at the door" and "hangs coat up in the closet after school." At school, if a student constantly blurts out incorrect answers in class, the target behaviour may be "waits 5 seconds before raising his hand to answer teacher's question." We often inadvertently reinforce impulsive behaviors of children by reacting too quickly.

Chart systems

A pioneer of behavioral psychology, Dr. Ogden Lindsley, had a motto which demonstrated his enthusiasm for using reinforcement principles in managing behaviour: *"Care enough to chart!"* By this, he meant that if parents (or teachers) take the time to target and monitor their charges' behaviour, they will often learn something important about the children, and will discover the means by which to positively influence their behaviour. Chart systems at home can be very useful in promoting cooperative behaviors, such as completing chores, doing homework and treating people in the household with courtesy and respect. Although several chore charts are commercially available, chart systems are only limited by your imagination and creativity.

Home-Based Point System

Behaviors to Increase (Points Earned)	Mon	Tue	Wed	Thur	Fri	Sat	Sun
Hangs up coat in closet & unloads backpack							
Checks Agenda & spends at least half hour doing homework before supper							
Etc.							
Etc.							
Behaviors to Decrease (Points Lost)							
Leaves supper table before finished or without permission							
Swears or talks back to parents							
Total Daily Points (Pts. Earned - Pts. Lost =)							

Token economies

The use of "token economies" or point systems have been described by psychologists Russell Barkley, William Pelham, Charles Cunningham and others. Dr. Barkley's *Taking Charge of ADHD* (updated 2005) is an excellent source for parents in developing positive reward charts at home, or home-school point systems. Also, Dr. Barkley's and Dr. Pelham's recommendations for using **Daily Report Cards** (DRCs) at school can be very effective in promoting on-task, cooperative and productive behaviors in school, with or without the benefit of stimulant medication. Of course, it takes some time and effort on the part of the teacher or teaching assistant to implement point programs for an individual student. However, the "pay-offs" in terms of classroom management are worth it. Often, teachers choose to have the entire class on some basic point program, which also benefits other special needs students. The points or tokens can be "cashed in" for special activity time or rewards at the end of the period, day or week. Additionally, parents and teachers may use the DRC as a method of school-home communication to monitor, recognize and reward their child's academic and behavioral progress in school. Daily report cards, based on three to five target behaviors, can also serve as an easy way to evaluate a student's response to medication changes or trials and other classroom interventions.

Daily (Behaviour) Report Card

Student will receive one point for demonstrating task or skill in each period. If student earns at least 8 points per day, then he gets a home reward:

Task/Skill	Lang. Arts before recess	Math after recess	Social/Science after lunch	Special Class Art, Music
Seatwork completed on time & with >80% accuracy				
Raises hand to answer/ask question				
Cooperates with class-mates				
Bonus: Follows recess & lunch rules		Name: _____		Date: _____
Total Daily Points		Teacher Signature: _____		

Punishment

Another main behaviour management principle is that negative consequences (or punishment) can have a suppressing effect on behaviour. However, there are dangers in using punishment (especially corporal punishment) as the only means of discipline, without having a positive parent-child relationship already established. If punitive measures are used routinely without any positive reinforcement of good behaviour, then the child only learns what he does wrong rather than what he can do to make things better. The child loses confidence in himself, becoming timid and fearful.

A note of caution here: Children should never be deprived of their regular meals, even when they are behaving badly, as good nutrition is important to the growth and learning of children.

The mildest form of punishment is actually the absence of any reinforcement, i.e., effectively ignoring misbehavior. Mildly disturbing behaviors, such as whining or temper tantrums ("hissy fits" to some), may be ignored as long as there is no risk of harm to the child or to others. Theoretically, an ignored behaviour will be reduced if everyone around the child withdraws his or her attention for a sufficient length of time. However, the negative behaviour often becomes worse before it gets better. A misbehaving child may try even harder to get people's attention, by resorting to more extreme behaviour and aggression if necessary. If a parent "gives in" and pays attention to the child during the outburst, then the child learns that extreme behaviour gets results. However, if a parent can "tough it out" and ignore the misbehavior long enough, then the child eventually gives up on the tactic of attempting to get a reaction from his parent.

Time-out

While there has been some difference of opinion about its appropriateness for discipline, "time out from positive reinforcement" is a structured way of withdrawing attention from a child. Time-out assumes that attention, or involvement in an activity, is reinforcing to the child. If the child is requested to "take a time-out" by removing himself from the situation, or sitting in a chair separate from the rest of the family or group for a few minutes, then whatever behaviour precipitated the call for time-out should be reduced in terms of its duration, intensity and frequency. A common rule of thumb is that one minute of time-out per year of age of the child is usually a sufficient length of time to calm down. If time-out does not reduce behaviour, after consistent use over several weeks, then it is not effective. Some kids misbehave in order to avoid doing difficult tasks or to get removed from the situation. Time-out may be more effective for pre-school and early elementary-aged children than older children. While time-out is a relatively mild form of punishment, and is much preferred over physical punishment, it should only be considered in the context of positive approaches to discipline. (The interested reader is directed to Dr. Thomas Phelan's 1995 book and videotape on *1, 2, 3 Magic*, a prescribed way of using time-out with young children. See suggested readings and websites.)

Russell Barkley, as well as Robert McMahon and Rex Forehand, have developed parenting programs to manage "defiant children" or "help the noncompliant child". Noncompliant, oppositional and defiant behaviour can become a major obstacle to cooperation and learning, both at home and in the classroom. These clinical researchers have demonstrated that a combination of providing clear requests (or "precision commands"), shaping compliant behaviour through positive reinforcement, and using brief time-out for blatant noncompliance can improve a young child's cooperation with adult requests. However, a noncompliant child's behaviour needs to be addressed well before the teenage years or there is a great risk of dangerous conduct problems developing, which are much more difficult to change.

Response Cost

Another mildly punishing technique, which may be especially helpful for impulsive children, is response cost. Response cost refers to the removal of a reward or privilege upon the commission of an undesired behaviour. "Grounding" from TV or video game privileges is a common example of response cost. Parents should be judicious in their use of grounding, as restricting a child from fun activities for too many days or weeks becomes a difficult punishment to enforce. Grounding for long periods of time can become discouraging to the child, who deserves to be given second or third chances to behave in better ways. It also can become a very unpleasant task to the enforcers of that punishment. Grounding should be time-limited and appropriate to the developmental age of the child.

The concept of response cost can also be used in token economies or point systems. If a child is earning points or tokens (poker chips, stickers or checkmarks on a chart) for good behaviour but then commits a thoughtless, impulsive act, a set number of points or tokens may be taken away from his point total. Losing points often causes impulsive children to "stop in their tracks" and consider a more reflective course of action. "Point loss" should only be introduced after a few weeks of implementing a positive point program. The impulsive child should still have opportunity to earn more points than he loses. If the child loses too many points and goes into a "deficit" position, then it can become very discouraging. Positive rein-forcement is meant to improve a child's motivation and self-esteem, as well as his behaviour.

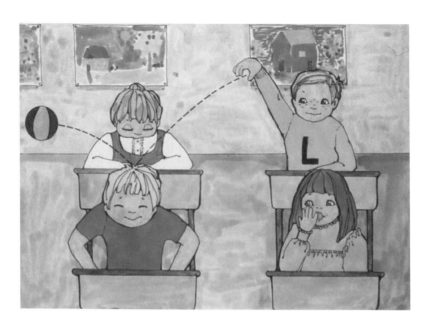

Cognitive Behaviour Therapy

In the 1970s and 1980s there was much interest in teaching cognitive behavioral strategies to children with ADHD and impulsive behaviour. Self-instructional training was promoted as a means to teach children to guide their own behaviour in more adaptive ways. Kendall and Braswell's cognitive behaviour therapy (CBT) program for impulsive children held much promise for training children, and their parents and teachers, in cognitive and social-emotional problem-solving techniques. Children with ADHD were capable of learning the CBT techniques in individual and group sessions with a clinician, especially when combined with a positive reward and response cost program. However, later research found that children did not continue to use these strategies on their own in home or classroom settings after the termination of treatment sessions. There was still a reliance on behaviour management techniques, as discussed previously, to maintain good behaviour in home, school and community settings. Nonetheless, the step-wise problem solving approach, that is central to most CBT, can be usefulwhen used collaboratively between children and their parents or teachers (see below).

Children with ADHD sometimes also have coexisting anxiety and/or mild depression. In these cases, CBT can be an effective, evidence-based psychosocial treatment for children to learn to cope with anxiety, change their negative thinking to a more positive outlook, and feel in control of their mood.

Collaborative Problem Solving

Another relatively new approach to child behaviour management is worth considering. Ross Greene, author of *The Explosive Child*, (second edition, 2001) has developed a form of parent and child therapy called Collaborative Problem Solving (CPS). Rather than providing positive or negative consequences *after* a behaviour, Dr. Greene suggests that parents (and teachers, too) can prevent non-compliant behaviour or explosive rages by using "teachable" moments *before* a behaviour escalates to the "point-of-no-return" or a "meltdown." That is, adults need to recognize that children with ADHD, and other chronic learning, behavioral, developmental and mood disorders lack the necessary skills to be successful in many daily tasks and activities. Because of deficits in the child's "executive function," language skills, and social-emotional competencies, etc., adults may need to "meet their children more than half-way" to help them develop the necessary cognitive and social-emotional skills to cope with daily frustrations. The CPS approach, which focuses on modifying the antecedents to misbehavior, attempts to change the conditions before a disruptive behaviour occurs so as to prevent it from happening. Proponents of CPS are currently trying to establish clinical and research evidence for this alternative approach to "manipulating" the rewarding or punishing consequences of behaviour.

Parenting Groups

How discipline techniques are most effectively communicated to parents has been the subject of much applied research over the past 20 or 30 years. Sound behavioral principles, presented in structured parenting classes or family management courses (for example, see Dallaire & Maunula, 1984), were not sufficient to create change in children's behaviour at home. During informational lectures, parents often seemed displeased with being treated as students who had much to learn from so-called "professionals." Also, parents felt that their unique challenges in parenting very difficult children were not being fully appreciated. They were often unwilling to try any suggested behavioral technique until they had opportunity to "tell their story" to a sympathetic audience. Recently, however, there has been an emphasis on using videotaped vignettes of parenting situations and "facilitated" group discussion as an effective way of promoting both knowledge and self-confidence in parents of difficult children (see for example, Carolyn Webster-Stratton's *Incredible Years* programs). Other parent education programs have recognized that parents, as a group, have a wealth of ideas and resources to be shared. Dr. Charles Cunningham and his colleagues in Hamilton, Ontario, have developed the **CO**mmunity **P**arent **E**ducation (COPE) program which is meant to be a school- or community-based, "family systems" approach to learning ways to effectively manage children's disruptive behaviour. A child's motivation and self-esteem, and positive couple and parent-child relationships, are emphasized as well as behavioral techniques. Community resources and social supports are also critical to parenting success in the COPE model.

When parent-training groups are offered through community- or hospital-based programs, it is important to also provide childcare through volunteer resources, as well as a social skills group for targeted children. Parenting groups must also recognize the need for self-care for a single parent or a couple who share the parenting duties. Besides parenting topics, ways to reduce stress and improve emotional regulation are explored in the group. A "*burnt-out*" parent will not be effective in raising competent children, no matter how many classes in behaviour management or discipline they attend. (Please see chapter 12 in R.A Barkley's book *Taking Charge at Home: The Art of Problem Solving* for an overview of Cunningham's problem-solving approach and other COPE program content.)

In conclusion, it should be noted that, "at the end of the day," there is no behavioral "magic pill" and that parenting or teaching a child can be a challenging and exhausting long-term task. However, it can be very much worth the effort in the long run. Children and adolescents with ADHD can learn to become happy, cooperative and productive adults when they have been given consistent guidance from their teachers and parents. Positive approaches to managing behaviour, by providing a balance of nurture and structure, can result in tremendous social-emotional growth and learning.

8   Classroom Management/ Educational Issues

Carol Skelly, MEd

The journey of a thousand miles begins with a single step.

Confucius circa 551-479 BC

It's the week before school starts in September. You have had a wonderful, restful summer and decide to spend some time preparing your classroom for your new students. In the hallway, you bump into the school resource teacher, who tells you that you will have only 20 students this year (good news) and two of them have been diagnosed with ADHD (bad news?). The resource teacher assures you that there will be a meeting early in September to discuss these students and to help you develop individual program plans (IPP). You suddenly decide to go home and finish the mystery that you started yesterday.

The first day of school rolls around and you see a small sea of twenty eager faces in Room 101. The girls and boys are dressed in neat looking outfits and many have new backpacks. As the children find seats on the carpet near your special "read aloud" chair, you notice a beautiful girl with golden angel hair, sitting near the edge of the rug. Her lovely blue eyes are staring dreamily out of the window and she is oblivious to the commotion around her. This is Angela. Across the room, a dark-haired stocky boy is shouting hello to his friends at the top of his voice. Then he punches and body checks others in his path to the carpet. "Hi, Ms R___," Dennis shouts in your face, as he collapses on the floor and rolls around. You check your watch to see how long it is until recess.

Sound somewhat familiar? At the risk of stereotyping ADHD students, many teachers would recognize Angela and Dennis. They would also be thrilled to have only 20 students in a class. However, the reality is that there are often other special needs students in much larger regular education classes – Layne, who has a learning disability; Bryan, who has behaviour difficulties; Gayle, who is gifted academically; Theo, who is a talented musician and Susan, who is shy and anxious. What's a teacher to do? How can a teacher meet the needs of all students in a regular class with minimal support and often few resources?

To repeat the maxim from the beginning of the chapter, "the journey of a thousand miles begins with a single step." The purpose of this chapter is to help teachers break the "problem" into smaller and more manageable chunks. By trying to meet the needs of Angela and Dennis, the ADHD students in Room 101, a teacher will often have the strategies to help all of the students in his or her class. Thoughtful, reflective teaching is great teaching, so let's reflect on how to support ADHD students in the regular education classroom.

First, reflect upon what you can change or adapt and what you cannot. You can change your attitude or perception of students. (Perhaps it is not bad news after all, to have Angela and Dennis in your class.) You can change your "tried and true" teaching methods, the classroom learning environment, the way you give feedback to parents, how you reinforce, motivate and assess your students. You *cannot* change your students' biological make-up, their parents or the weather. Clearly, there are many more areas that you can change. The following suggestions may help in your teaching/learning journey that feels like a thousand miles in September but is really only ten short months. These ten months can have a significant, positive impact on your students and on you.

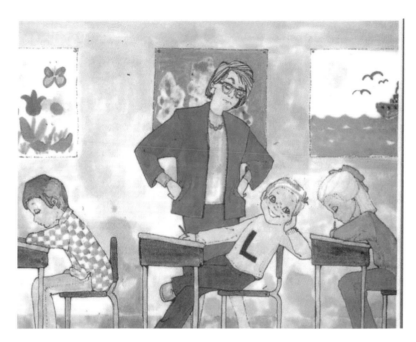

Relationships/Rapport/Connections

The first and most important point to reflect upon is *who* your students are. While there are commonalities among ADHD students, they are all individuals. Angela is very different from Dennis. Knowing your students' strengths, needs and histories can be a major first step in developing an appropriate educational plan. Here are some questions to guide your reflection:

- How old is the student? When is his/her birth date? Are they young for their grade placement? This can be a more significant issue for boys than girls in terms of language and social skills.

- Have they been retained? This can have a negative effect on their academic self-esteem and may be a red flag for subtle learning problems.

- Are there other issues impacting on learning? Does the student have sensory problems – vision and /or hearing loss; learning disabilities, and/or behaviour problems? ADHD students have higher rates of learning problems, anxiety/emotional problems, and/or behaviour/conduct difficulties beyond the typical ADHD problems of inattention, impulsivity and/or hyperactivity. This is called co-morbidity, i.e., when other issues coexist with ADHD.

- What are their preferred learning styles: visual, auditory, tactile and/or kinesthetic?

- Where do they fit in terms of Gardner's multiple intelligence model: verbal/linguistic, musical/rhythmic, logical/mathematical, visual/spatial, bodily/kinesthetic, naturalist, intrapersonal, interpersonal?

- Is there a family history of learning and attention problems (parents and older siblings)?

The next point to reflect upon is *who* you are as a teacher. Are you a calm, orderly person, who needs a great deal of structure in the classroom? Are you an enthusiastic exciting teacher with a high tolerance for noise and chaos in the classroom? Interestingly, many ADHD students are a better match with the former type teacher, but they behave like the latter.

When you understand yourself and your teaching style, then you are in a better position to try to accommodate to the needs of ADHD students in your class. Remember earlier in this chapter, there was a mention of what you can change and what you cannot. It is much more realistic to change yourself than others. The hope would be that your changes or adaptations would positively shape the behaviour of your students. Isn't that what teaching comes down to – shaping behaviour in a positive way? What a challenge and a responsibility!

Yes, it is a tremendous challenge to like a difficult student when you have so many other students who need your attention. But if the student perceives that you do not see him as a problem but as a child with a problem, he will likely try harder in his struggle to cope with his problem. Rekindling hope in his struggling heart to be as successful as his peers is a key to progress and, in turn, very rewarding for you. Then the very important issue of rapport or relationship building can be addressed.

ADHD is a biological condition and thus these students are not out to "get you" or to ruin your perfect classroom. (Does such a thing exist?) ADHD students want to do well and aim to please, but they "leap before they look." Think of *Dennis the Menace*. They can be warm, creative, affectionate students, who just happen to drive you insane on a Friday afternoon. (See the list at the end of this chapter – 25 good things about ADHD.) If you can build a positive connection with these students, it can be a tremendous support for their battered self-esteem. Often, ADHD students receive many negative messages at school, from peers, teachers, bus drivers and others, that they are "bad" kids. If you can focus on prevention (anticipating problems during transitions, catching them when they are "good") and provide supportive accommodations (assigning a study buddy, allowing preferential seating), then life in your classroom will run more smoothly for you and all of your students.

School is hard work for special needs students, like those with ADHD and/or learning disabilities. They need many more positive comments and experiences to offset the huge number of negatives they get in the school hallways, the neighborhood streets and sometimes their homes. Resilient students have commented that having a significant and positive adult in their lives made all the difference. You are that significant person.

Learning Environment

There is one aspect of the teaching/learning scenario that is fairly easy to adapt and that is the learning environment. The classroom can be quite easily modified to better meet the needs of ADHD students, and often, all students. As mentioned in the last section, preferential seating is a key issue. Seating Angela or Dennis close to the source of instruction, (i.e., the teacher, the overhead projector, and the whiteboard), and away from visual and auditory distractions, such as the windows, the door to the hallway, the noisy heating vent, is highly recommended. It is very instructive for teachers to sit and observe students, if possible (called "kidwatching" by Yetta Goodman). This observation of the student within the learning environment is helpful for the teacher to get a "kid's eye view" of the situation. What are factors that might be distracting? Is the desk/table at the correct height? Is the chair comfortable? Are the written instructions clear and readable from where the student sits? Are the students surrounding the ADHD child distracters or helpers? Is the student's desk disorganized?

Teachers lose a lot of valuable information when they are teaching at the front of the room rather than observing from the back. Observing the class while another person teaches is a particularly valuable experience, as is videotaping your instruction (for those who are brave). Seating the ADHD student beside a good role model/study buddy is potentially a good idea, as long as the high performing student is willing and not bothered by this extra responsibility. This would give the ADHD child a chance to check oral instructions and see how a good student works. It may prevent some procrastination due to lack of understanding of what to do. Some ADHD students have found a "Move & Sit" cushion helpful. This cushion forces the student to continually try to keep the core of their body stable and thus provides physical stimulation without disturbing others around them (available from www.fitter1.com).

Keeping the classroom calm and quiet by minimizing noise helps ADHD students attend better. Classrooms can be amazingly noisy environments but teachers are often unaware of the many distracting noises (chairs dragging on bare floors, low level talking, bells ringing, overhead announcements) because they are so busy teaching. Some teachers put slit tennis balls on the legs of desks and chairs to reduce noise. Carpets can soften noise. ADHD students who are easily distracted by sounds may need to wear noise abating headphones to shut out noise. Study carrels or large cardboard boxes can be used as "offices" for visually distracted students. It is important to conceptualize this "office space" as a privilege and not a punishment. Allowing top students to use the "office" as well, is a good idea. Some classrooms are too busy visually. Teachers are masters at decorating their rooms beautifully. Perhaps less is more where ADHD students are concerned, especially if visual distractions are a problem.

Many instructional tools like computers, tape recorders, FM systems, and stress or squeeze balls can make the classroom environment more user-friendly for ADHD students. The sky is the limit in terms of creative reconfiguration of the classroom environment. The only limit would be the teacher's imagination and the support of the school principal and custodian.

Teaching Tips/Instructional Strategies

Teaching is a life-long learning process – the longer you have taught and the more students you have connected with, the more teaching strategies you may have added to your repertoire. But even better, is if you and other teachers in your school support each other by sharing tips about coping with ADHD students. That is the intention of this chapter – one experienced teacher sharing ideas with others. Of course not all strategies work with all students because Angela is very different from Dennis. ADHD students are individuals with different interests, strengths and needs. However, some strategies do address the most common difficulties experienced by ADHD students.

Attention

Attention is a key factor in learning. Getting and keeping a student's attention means that the child will benefit more from the teacher's instruction. Let's call this optimal performance or an ideal situation. We know, as teachers, that all students lose their focus at times due to fatigue, hunger, worry or fear. Children with ADHD, however, lose their focus more often than does the average student. Cue the inattentive student verbally, visually or by touch. Stand next to the student when giving instructions. Check that the child understands and has "heard" the directions. Make eye contact. Combine visual and auditory information. Give directions orally and then write the key points on the board. Break down the instructions into manageable portions for the ADHD student, so that the student remains focused and is not overwhelmed with too much information at a time.

Hyperactivity

Hyperactivity is another hallmark of ADHD students and movement breaks are a good solution for this difficulty. Allowing these children socially acceptable opportunities to get up from their seat, stretch and move around will help to prevent more aimless wandering around the classroom. Being sensitive to the need to move as a way for ADHD kids to stimulate themselves and keep focused is important. Also, teachers need to be aware of the low tolerance that ADHD students have for boring repetitive tasks and to try to increase the interest factor or at least keep lessons short and sweet. Have Dennis demonstrate a Math example on the overhead projector with coloured pens. Ask Angela to carry a note to the office and have a drink of water on the way back as a reward for time on task.

Impulsivity

Impulsivity is another common trait of students with ADHD. Help these students to s-l-o-w d-o-w-n. Keep instructions short and simple (K.I.S.S.). Repeat instructions as needed. It is pointless and frustrating to tell an ADHD student, "I just told you that." If he had heard the instructions properly, the student would not be asking for clarification. Actually asking for clarification is an excellent strategy that should be praised. In fact, a student asking for clarification is a more active learner than one who does not know how to proceed but does not ask for a variety of reasons (lack of self monitoring, fear of humiliation). It also is a red flag for the teacher that this child has some difficulties that need attention.

Show Angela how to chunk her work and complete one short section rather than be overwhelmed by a whole page. Ask Dennis to talk through the steps of an activity or problem before he begins a task. Provide immediate feedback as soon and as often as possible. Perhaps fold a Math sheet into four or six sections. Then mark each section. This also prevents the student from overlearning any errors.

Probably the best instructional strategy is to teach problem-solving skills across the curriculum, including the social-emotional area. Many ADHD students act first and think later (*impulsivity*). A problem solving approach reverses this sequence by emphasizing a "think first, act later" style of doing things. One of the simplest and most effective problem solving methods is the use of the following questions. (Some teachers include visual cues for younger students – a stop sign shape, a light bulb, arrows, green and red traffic lights.) Teaching a "stop and think" problem-solving strategy requires the teacher to model how to do this. Modeling and repetition are very powerful in student learning.

- What is the problem?   STOP
- Focus. Pay attention.   SELF-TALK
- What is the best plan?   THINK
- Try it.   ACT
- Did the plan work?   EVALUATE
- How did I do?   SELF-MONITOR
- Try again (if it did not work).   ACT

Another important teaching strategy is positive and specific praise. Teachers often use praise to motivate students. However, ADHD students do not always get enough praise because their behaviour may attract more negative attention than positive. The challenge for the teacher is to ensure that the positive comments outweigh the negatives by being very self-reflective about the verbal (and non-verbal) feedback given. Try to make a mental note that for every "negative" comment to Dennis ("sit down") or to Angela ("sit up") that you provide three to five "positives." Finally, the best teachers for ADHD students seem to be calm, clear and consistent individuals. Direct instruction works well with students like Angela and Dennis. Open-ended activities and group work can be difficult for ADHD kids, as they have problems with self-regulation and executive functioning. They need guidance and guidelines – in other words, provide structure.

Study Skills/Organization/Testing

Many ADHD students are described as disorganized. This makes perfect sense, as these young people are impulsive and inattentive. By definition, an organized person is good at planning and self-reflection (these are executive functioning abilities). Some professionals have called ADHD a disorder in the area of executive functioning. So how do teachers get their "mini-executives" to function better? As hiring a personal secretary (or teaching assistant) for each ADHD student in the class is not feasible, the next best solution is to directly teach and actively reinforce good organizational/study skills.

Teachers, especially high school teachers, expect students to come to school with well-developed skills in this area. The reality is that this is not the case for most students and especially ADHD kids. Therefore, time spent teaching adolescents and even younger students how to "get organized," is time well spent. There are numerous materials in the public library or bookstores on this topic. Here are a few areas that need special attention for students with "attention" problems.

1.   Time at the end of the day/class to write down what they are expected to do for homework. Have this written in a concise but clear manner so that parents have an idea about the teachers' expectations. (Due dates, whether the assignment can be handwritten or typed, etc.) In some cases, the teacher will need to sign the organizers of a few students to emphasize the importance of this task. While signing, the teacher may remind the ADHD student to pack the correct textbooks and/or notebooks needed to do their homework. If this becomes a major problem, then a spare set of texts could be sent home (if possible).

2.   Remember the purpose of homework. It is not to have students tackle new work but to reinforce concepts learned in school. ADHD students on medication may be at a distinct disadvantage doing homework, if the benefit of the medication has worn off. Check with the parents periodically (in the agenda) to see how long it takes to complete the homework or if there are significant battles getting homework completed. Consider reducing the amount of work done at home to the most necessary or beneficial activities.

3. Help ADHD (and all) students learn how to break down large projects into smaller, more manageable chunks with short-term deadlines, using an outline or project guide. Completing major projects on time is a tough skill to learn even for university students and especially for ADHD individuals.

4. Teach ADHD students how to take tests strategically. Skim over the test first, then go back and answer the easy questions first. Then read the hard questions very carefully (for the third time) to ensure that the student has not misread the question. Impulsive and inattentive students often read too quickly and thus answer a "different" question than is on the test page. Encourage the students to check their work to avoid careless errors, especially in Math. The teacher can model good test-taking skills.

5. Allow ADHD students to have special exam adaptations. The two most helpful accommodations are extra time and a quiet distraction-free space to write the exam. Many departments of education allow this, even for significant exams at the end of the year. Some documentation to prove that the student indeed has a true attention deficit/hyperactivity disorder may be required.

6. In some cases, if a learning disability is present along with ADHD, then the student should have access to a computer to write exams. As well, he could have tests, read aloud (or on tape) and answers scribed by an adult.

7. Provide study guides and clear expectations for what material will be tested. Teach memory tricks (mnemonics) to help students remember facts. (For example, H.O.M.E.S. is an acronym for the Great Lakes in Canada – **H**uron, **O**ntario, **M**ichigan, **E**rie, **S**uperior.) Use index cards for vocabulary study or for Math proce-

dures (the steps in a Math operation) or discrete facts (addition, multiplication, history, science).

8.   Do not rely on just one test, but rather on multiple assessment tools (observation, informal measures of the learning process and product) to gain a true picture of the ADHD (and all) students' strengths and needs. If there are problems, *re-teach*.

9.   Finally, use tests as a teaching tool. Review what the student does not know/remember. Allowing re-tests is a true learning experience. Have students teach each other. The best way to learn something is to teach another.

The Journey Continues

June 28th. The students have packed up all their books, artwork and projects. After the end of year party mess is cleaned up, with Angela and Dennis' help, you collapse into your reading chair and have a look at the card that the entire class signed. How many steps have been taken in this journey of a year?

Angela has started to truly bloom and is becoming a very helpful child. Her self-esteem has improved dramatically. It is still necessary to get her attention very purposefully during a lesson but Angie does well when she knows what to do. She is such a bright child.

Dennis has struggled with paying attention and staying in his seat. Recently, he went back to see his pediatrician to have his stimulant medication reviewed. The doctor asked that some forms be completed to learn how Dennis behaves and attends in class. New medication was tried that really seemed to help this boy cope better in the regular class. Dennis can be so funny and endearing when he is not racing around the room distracting other students. You make a mental note to put Dennis in a class next year with a teacher who has a kind but structured approach to behaviour management. All in all, a wonderful year with great kids, even the two "bad news" students, who turned out to be "good news" after all.

The following list was generated by the children, parents and the staff of an ADD camp organized by the Calgary Learning Centre in the summer of 1992. The experience was very moving for both the parents and their children because it helped them look beyond the negative implications associated with ADHD to identify the positive characteristics.

1. Lots of energy.

2. Willing to try things- takes risk.

3. Ready to talk, can talk a lot.

4. Gets along well with adults.

5. Can do several things at one time.

6. Smart.

7. Needs less sleep.

8. Good sense of humor.

9. Very good at taking care of younger kids.

10. Spontaneous.

11. Sees detail that other people miss.

12. Understands what it is like to be teased or to be in trouble, so is understanding of other kids.

13. Can think of different and new ways to do things.

14. Volunteers to help others.

15. Happy and enthusiastic.

16. Imaginative – creative.

17. Articulate – can say things well.

18. Sensitive – compassionate.

19. Eager to make new friends.

20. Great memory.

21. Courageous.

22. More fun to be with than most kids.

23. Charming.

24. Warm and loving.

25. Cares a lot about families.

Obviously not every ADHD child possesses all of these positive qualities. However, every ADHD child has some of these qualities to help him be successful and to help make teaching him a rewarding experience for the teacher.

9   Parenting and Family Life

Mila Wendt, MSW

Character cannot be developed in ease and quiet. Only through experience of trial and suffering can the soul be strengthened, ambition inspired, and success achieved.

Helen Keller 1880-1968

Parenting is difficult. In all probability parenting has always been difficult. Perhaps every generation of parents has felt that their task has been the most challenging. Parenting, at the best of times, is an incredible and humbling responsibility. Even parenting "easy" children in ordinary family situations can be hard. Parenting of a child with special needs, of whatever sort, is even more demanding. And when family life is complicated, for whatever other reasons (such as parental illness, financial strain, divorce, etc.), and a child has special needs, the challenges become tougher. Also, we know that children with ADHD often have parents who have ADHD, which again multiplies the challenges. Parenting a child with ADHD can be a very challenging task that requires patience and courage. By far the vast majority of parents of ADHD children manage to meet the challenge and successfully raise their family.

Impact of the Diagnosis

Parental reaction to the diagnosis of ADHD varies from family to family. It may take time to come to an understanding or acceptance. Whatever the many emotions you may experience as you deal with the diagnosis of ADHD, allow yourself to have your feelings without criticizing or blaming yourself. You may have felt that from an early age your child was "different." Relatives, friends, or neighbours may have suggested that your child's annoying behaviors were due to your poor parenting. Perhaps you have been living without answers for years, having your concerns down-played by others, not knowing or understanding what is happening to your child and your family, and so hearing the diagnosis of ADHD may be a relief. Having a name for your child's difficulties, a way to make sense of the differences and struggles, and strategies to put in place, may make all the difference in your world. You may see the diagnosis as an opportunity to make your child's life better. Or, you may find out when your child is very young, and wonder if the diagnosis is really correct. Some families find out gradually, from their own suspicions and reading, and then receiving a professional confirmation. Then again, facing the reality of an ADHD diagnosis may be extremely painful and something that takes you a long while to understand and accept. You and your partner may differ in your understanding and acceptance of the disorder, especially if one parent has more daily contact with the child and is more involved in attending appointments.

However you and your child come to the diagnosis of ADHD, it has probably been a voyage of discovery. Often, parents need to take things slowly in dealing with such a diagnosis. You may want to take time to ask questions, to absorb the answers, and to ask more questions. You may be angry and want to find something or someone to blame. There may be disbelief and denial of the existence of the disorder, of the accuracy of the diagnosis, of the competency of the involved professionals. You may feel guilty, insecure, or experience a sense of failure. You may question "Why did this happen to us?" It is natural for parents to experience sadness, or even grief, when they are told that their child has ADHD. Rest assured, however, that while raising a child with ADHD can be an enormous challenge, it is not a disaster. It is likely to be an adventure, and it may even be fun. Changing, and even having to give up, some of your hopes about the pleasure of raising your family and the future of your children can feel like a loss. All parents have dreams for their children, and our vision of "the ideal life" for them may be challenged by the reality of the struggles ahead. Most parents meet these challenges and many of them are surprised when their ADHD child becomes successful and productive as an adult, even beyond their original dreams.

It is important to have a balanced picture. Having ADHD, and receiving the diagnosis, is not a calamity. There is a positive side to ADHD. This disorder brings its own gifts into our lives. People with ADHD are often creative, candid, fun, spontaneous, outgoing, energetic, interesting, innovative, spirited, compassionate, curious, charming and loving. The list goes on. They can be good at multi-tasking, taking risks, and thinking "out of the box." They can demonstrate a great memory for, and persistence (even tenacity) with, the things that interest them. In fact, some of the very things that can make a child with ADHD a challenge to raise may be great assets in adulthood. As you see the positive traits associated with ADHD, you can help your child to appreciate his own unique talents. Seeing the diagnosis of ADHD as an opportunity, rather than a burden, will assist your child to develop a positive self-image and a stronger sense of self.

Resources

Finding, obtaining and maintaining resources and services for your child (and family) can be a major responsibility and challenge for parents. Services may be in short supply, there may be gaps in services, waiting lists may be long, and financial costs may be a barrier. Because these obstacles may be present when parents seek professional referrals or specialized resources, being your child's advocate is an essential role. This can also be an emotionally taxing process.

You may feel that, at times, your physician does not appreciate the depth of your family's distress. You may feel dismissed or not heard. It may be painful to discuss family difficulties. Telling your story over and over again, to yet another professional, may be draining and frustrating. As parents, it is natural to identify with your children's pain and struggles, and depending on the strength of that identification and your sense of injustice, it may be difficult to not overreact or be defensive. It is in your child's best interest if a working alliance can be developed with the professionals involved in his care. This may require some extra effort on your part, but can pay great dividends. Some of the following strategies might be helpful:

- Prepare to meet a professional by writing down specific goals, concerns or questions that you want to address and bring them to the meeting. Taking notes at the meeting can also be helpful.

- Allow the professional to address your concerns, one at a time.

- Adopt a listening attitude, being as open-minded and flexible as possible.

- Feel free to ask questions and clarify points you do not understand.

There are a number of resources that you may find useful. You may want help understanding more about ADHD, or to talk to someone in-depth regarding your worries about your child's problematic behaviors. Or perhaps you are having trouble with coping and need a listening ear and some guidance. Maybe you want to improve family communication or strengthen your child's self esteem. Family therapy, parental counselling or coaching, parent education workshops, behaviour management, parenting groups and social skill groups are some approaches that you may want to consider. Many can be accessed through your family doctor, your child's school, a local community centre or community health services.

Professionally-led parenting groups that meet over time and focus on learning and/or skill development can be of great assistance. They offer the opportunity to discuss feelings, problems, strategies and solutions with others who are experiencing similar difficulties. Parent groups can help you to identify and clarify issues, as well as develop, implement, practice, and evaluate other strategies to deal with your concerns. Though attending an ongoing group can be intimidating, many parents have reported experiencing a sense of validation and safety from other group members, which supported their learning and a process of change. Knowing that you are not alone, that there are other parents and children who can relate to what you are going through, who have felt as you do, who share your sense of struggle or pain, can be an immense relief.

Self-help parent support groups can be a lifeline. CHADD (Children and Adults with ADHD) is a nation wide non-profit support group, available in many cities and via the Internet, which can be a valuable source of information and assistance. See their website at the end of this book.

When More is Needed

If, despite your efforts, a negative cycle develops, family members feel diminished. As family harmony is reduced, you may unintentionally take your pain out on each other. You may also avoid each other, and disagreements may go unattended and fester. Normal differences of opinions may feel overwhelming. Instead of a place of safety and comfort, your family may feel chaotic and toxic. Family breakdown may occur, leaving everyone feeling devastated. If your marriage or family is also struggling with other serious issues (addictions, violence, trauma, physical or mental illness, job loss, etc), the added stress and demands of an ADHD child may temporarily overwhelm your available resources. Some parents may reach a point where they are at risk of harming themselves, each other or their child, emotionally and/or physically. If this is the case for you, consider reaching out for professional help immediately. Your doctor, a help line or hospital emergency department can direct you further. Most families with an ADHD child do not face these extreme difficulties. Do not despair. Help is on hand. Read on.

Surviving, Coping, Thriving

Given that there is no set path, how do families navigate their experiences? Though you may share some commonalities and experiences with others, every child, every parent, every family impacted by ADHD is unique.

Feeling Overwhelmed

As a parent of an ADHD child you can experience a great deal more disappointment, frustration, confusion and discouragement than with your other children. There can be a sense of stigma, shame and isolation. At times, every member of the family may feel hurt, angry and misunderstood. Little by little, conflict might extend to all areas of family life and it may seem that peace of mind is elusive. Somehow, despite your best intentions, continuous crisis may become a way of life. Success may be rare and you may come to expect the worse, dreading every phone call. This kind of constant stress can take an emotional toll. Some parents describe feeling burdened, trapped, helpless, hopeless and defeated. You may struggle with a sense of inadequacy. You may feel such a weight on your shoulders (or your heart) that you never before thought possible. Fatigue can set in and you feel drained. As negative behaviors escalate despite your best efforts, and blame and self-blame increase, you may regularly experience shame, humiliation and even rage. How does a family steer around or break out of such a position?

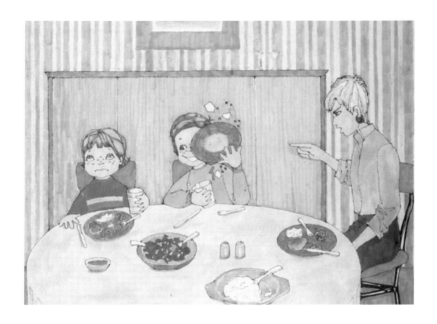

When life is so difficult, how do you help yourself, and each other?

The Value of Learning about ADHD

Inform yourself. Educating yourself about ADHD and its management is one of the most important things you can do. Use your newly acquired knowledge and advisors to assist and support you, in your job and responsibilities as a parent. You may encounter skepticism about the diagnosis of ADHD or hear frightening stories about medication. The decision about using medication can be a difficult one. Parents have many questions, such as: "What is ADHD?" "Is ADHD a fad?" "Will my child grow out of ADHD?" "How do I discipline if I am not sure what is ADHD and what is just plain misbehavior?" "Isn't my child just being stubborn or wanting his own way?" "How do I answer my mother (father, in-laws, relatives, neighbors, etc) when they say he just needs a good spanking?"

As a parent it is important to know, for instance, that ADHD is a biologically caused disorder. It is an identifiable and treatable condition and is not caused by "poor" parenting. Knowledge will help you to answer some of your questions and to figure out where to go to ask the other questions. Knowledge can prevent an unnecessary cycle of self-blame, and criticism. There are now many sources of information: books, articles, the Internet and the media. There is a list at the back of this book that can get you started. You need, however, to be skeptical and vigilant about the accuracy or quality of that information. The old adage "Don't believe everything you hear" can prove to be excellent advice. Look for "evidence based" information (backed by credible research) and trustworthy sources (the reference list at the back of this book is a good foundation).

Awareness

This includes self-awareness, as well as being aware of the impact of ADHD on others. How are your expectations of parenting, of what your child "should" accomplish, of how his life will turn out, etc., affecting your choices and behaviour? Consider what the impact of having a child with ADHD is on you, on your partner, on your other children, on the family as a whole. Do you or does your partner have ADHD/ADD? Or are you beginning to suspect this might be the case?

Impact on Self

Coping with a child who has ADHD can be exhausting. Pay attention to your own well-being, your own health and energy. You may be feeling over-burdened by your responsibilities. Though it is hard, making the effort to find time for you will likely have positive results in the end. You will be better able to care for your child and meet his needs if you feel energetic, rest-ed, competent and worthwhile. Getting, and keeping, a positive sense of well-being will be a difficult task in itself, especially when it hurts to witness your child's struggles. Some basic guidelines can be helpful: Exercise regularly. Eat a well balanced diet including plenty of fresh fruits and vegetables. Drink lots of water. Strive to maintain a weight that is healthy for your body type. Get enough sleep. Have fun on a regular basis, laugh, and practice relaxation (deep breathing, yoga, prayer, meditation, visualization, positive thinking, the options are many). Develop a spiritual life according to your own belief system and make time for friends and your personal interests.

Impact on Marriage

As a child with ADHD requires more of your time than your other children do, it may be hard to ensure that your other children and your partner do not feel neglected. If you are in a marriage, it is vital to preserve and nurture your adult relationship. Be aware that the demands of a child with ADHD may take a toll on your relationship and take what steps you can to appreciate and strengthen your bonds. Enjoy whatever shared vacations you can, even half hour ones. Recognize that strains on your marriage are to be expected. Avoid over-involvement or over-focusing on the ADHD child. Share responsibilities and actively co-parent, if you can. It is not unusual for parents to differ in how they view things. No two parents agree 100 percent of the time; you may even see your partner as overly harsh or indulgent. But it is critical that you and your partner learn to handle conflict and disagreement constructively, as there will be plenty of it. It is important to address conflicts, rather than avoiding arguments out of fear. Take care to keep adult issues separate from the children's issues. Regularly evaluate the success of your parenting approaches with your partner in private. Respectful listening, goodwill, demonstrating concern and empathy, and an open mind will increase success. And as always, patience is helpful. Successful problem resolution is a skill that your children will benefit from, especially if they have the opportunity to observe you practicing it on a regular basis.

Impact on Parenting

When continually challenged by your ADHD child, you may lose perspective and start to doubt your own parenting skills. Know that you are not to blame, and in fact you are an important part of the "treatment." It may be hard to remain loving, understanding, patient and calm especially in the face of provocative behaviour. Knowing the difference between your child's lack of skill in the moment and non-compliance will sometimes be tough. Your child needs you to be the competent adult, the authority, the source of strength, even as he taxes your patience. He needs you to be strong enough not to be shaken by his testing behaviors. As parents, we have a great deal of influence over our children. How we respond to our children, not just in the good times, but also the challenging times, will help to shape the person they will become. Although it can be tempting to temporarily abandon your parental role, and to give in or give up, it is not in your child's best interest to do so. Keep talking (with your partner, your friends, a therapist) and resist blaming others. Seek out support to maintain (or regain) your confidence. Keep in mind that your child has a biological disorder. His ADHD behaviors are not intentional and are not purposefully designed to anger you, though it may seem like that at times. Try to see your child's actions as due to his attentional difficulties or impulsivity and not due to his being bad. Structure his environment to encourage and support the behaviour you desire. Understanding and remembering that your child will probably have difficulties with self-control, delaying gratification, and remembering instructions, will help you to keep your expectations reasonable. Use self-calming strategies when needed (deep breathing, non-escalating thoughts, etc.). Try not to perceive your child's misbehavior as a threat to your credibility as a parent, but rather see it as an expression of his struggle in learning life's tough lessons. Dealing well with these parental challenges, successfully assisting your child, helping him find the hidden "treasure" of his strengths, can be rewarding and bring tremendous satisfaction.

You and your child's other parent may be separated or divorced and this can make a challenging situation even more difficult. If at all possible, in the best interests of all involved children, seek to establish and maintain an amicable, respectful parenting relationship with your "ex." Be conscious of appropriate adult–child boundaries and strive to keep adult matters between the adults. Be aware of the damage that putting the children in the middle can do. If there is no support or involvement forthcoming, then caring for yourself and building a community of support for you and your child are very important. If there are no family support groups in your community, talk with your friends and neighbors and start a group. Parents can learn a lot from each other.

Impact on Family Life

ADHD affects the entire family, not just the child with ADHD. Keeping the family "climate" stable, despite the constant "storms" of the ADHD child can be quite a challenge. It is important to do what you can to structure your home environment to encourage, if not harmony and peace, at least some sense of calm. Positive emotional states are good for our health. Your attitude of hope and optimism (or not) can have a ripple effect through the family. As the adult, if you know that a change in the family climate is needed, the leadership position to initiate change is yours. Cultivate, from small seeds if necessary, connectedness and a family sense of belonging. Acknowledge and celebrate small successes. Think of positive human contact as preventive maintenance. Given the conflicts that will inevitably arise, it is vital that positive family interactions are encouraged. Self care, nurturing interactions, paying attention to the little things in each other's lives, making time for one another on a daily basis, cooking and eating together, or sharing adventures might be ways to bolster a sense of connectedness in your family. Attending a parent support group or family therapy might be options to consider, as well.

Impact on Siblings

Your child's brothers and sisters will need your attention and nurturing too. They may resent their sib with ADHD, and the time given to him, and may need your guidance on how to deal with these strong feelings. It can be difficult to modify your expectations of your ADHD child, and still feel that you are being fair to the others. When one child seems to need, even demand, so much adult energy, you may wonder how you can also remember and attend to the needs of the other children. Sibs may fall into the destructive habit of blaming the child with ADHD for everything. Also, if you have more than one child with ADHD, sibling interactions can be more intense. These dynamics become even more complex when siblings have other special needs of their own. Yet, finding the time to value each child for who he is, is a critical task of parenting.

Impact on the Child

Your child needs your help to understand and believe that ADHD is not "bad," but rather a "difference." It is critical to establish and maintain an open, friendly relationship with your child. Your child needs your reassurance that they have done nothing wrong to have ADHD and that you love him. His anger and frustration, his inability to appreciate the impact of his behaviour on others, his rejection by peers can make his daily life a minefield to negotiate. Help your child feel safe by knowing nothing can shake your love for them. When he is frustrated and discouraged, he needs to know that even if he has given up hope (for the moment), you have not. Hope is one of the most powerful attitudes that you can model for your child. Help him discover what he likes to do, and what he is good at doing. Convey your belief that he will succeed, in his own way and in his own time. Help him find social and recreational activities where he can succeed, feel a sense of mastery and competency, and so develop self-esteem.

Dealing with Others

Other people, from your parents to your neighbors, may not always agree with your approach, and may feel free to express their disapproval or to criticize you or your child. They may give you unsolicited and, at times, conflicting advice. You may feel angry, defensive and blamed personally for your child's misbehavior. It may help to remember that your neighbors, your extended family, even professionals, do not have all of the information that you have. Certainly they have not experienced what you have been through. So it is not surprising if there is a gap in their appreciation and understanding of your position. It may be hard not to harbor resentment against others for their negative judgments, so try to find a safe place to share your intense feelings, so that you can let them go. Do not allow their comments and suggestions to make you feel that you are inadequate as a parent or your child's behaviour is due to your poor parenting skills. Remind them, and yourself, that you have other well-behaved children.

Coping

Yes, you and your family can survive. You can learn to cope successfully, and you can also discover how to thrive! Instead of viewing ADHD as a catastrophe, you may see it, at some point down the road, as a blessing that has enriched your life. How do you empower yourself as a parent so as to provide optimal care for often-challenging children, as well as caring for other family members and the family as a whole? What is helpful in this process? Certainly education about ADHD and self-awareness is helpful. And there are a number of other principles that can guide you on your voyage of discovery.

A Focus on Hope and Strengths

As mentioned earlier, hope (and optimism) is critical. Children with ADHD often have a unique way of looking at the world. This special way of being (creative, spontaneous, energetic, etc.) and their resilience can be celebrated as gifts. Centering your parenting on your values and beliefs is vital. Keeping yourself healthy (emotionally and physically), and grounded in your family and community is important. Nurturing relationships, connectedness and positive interactions can go a long way to reducing stress. A focus on your own and your child's strengths is helpful. This includes identifying, remembering, valuing and keeping strengths in the front-and-centre of your attention. Using your own competencies and looking for the competency of your child ("catch him/her being good") is important. Establishing a loving family life where children learn first hand about trust and stability is helpful. Having adult relationships (marital or otherwise) that model constructive problem-solving and respectful conflict resolution is indispensable.

Emotional Regulation

Emotional regulation, a goal for all of us, becomes even more critical for the family dealing with ADHD. It is important, as a parent, to model emotional self-regulation if your wish is for your child to learn to subordinate his impulses to the values you are trying to teach. In order to help our children learn emotional regulation we must do so ourselves. Yet, it can be difficult to keep your own "cool" in the face of your child's provocative behaviour and family volatility. Words are powerful and your child needs encouraging words from you, even when you may be tempted to use inappropriate words in frustration. Learn how to express your disapproval without attacking your child's character. Make it clear, that even when you are following through with consequences, you are acting out of love and respect for them. Consequences should be established and carried out in an environment of unqualified love and mutual respect and should convey the lesson that you intend to teach. Beware of the negative cycle of exerting greater and greater punitive control over your child. Great patience, and even outside support, may be necessary. How you balance nurturing and discipline in a consistent, predictable environment can have a powerful impact. Yet, know that nobody expects you to be perfect; it is how you respond most of the time that matters.

Understanding Your Child's Point of View

Striving to appreciate your child's perspective will help to foster a climate of trust and understanding. Though it may be hard, work at understanding where your child is coming from, and why he is behaving, from his point of view, the way he is. "Walking a mile in his shoes" can help you stay in touch with your compassionate side when you are frustrated with your child's behaviour. Consider if your child feels listened to, and be prepared to listen every day, offering encouragement and support despite all of the problems. Seek first to understand your child, and only then, to have him understand your position. Probably, it is not that your child is deliberately pushing your buttons, but rather that he is frustrated by what is expected of him and does not know how to appropriately express his frustration. It is not your child's fault that he has ADHD. Though you may be confused by his behaviour, this may be how the world makes sense to him at this point in time. Knowing that you are "in his/her corner" is invaluable to your child. There are many ways you can convey this: paying attention, empathic listening, being interested in his world, respecting and/or validating his point of view even when you might not agree, spending time together, having fun together, sharing laughter, etc.

Consistent, United Parenting

Establishing parental credibility is important, as is your own confidence in your parenting. Consistent, united parenting, that is, working as a team, agreeing upon rules, expectations, and structure, and following through, increases the chance of success in influencing a child's behaviour. Ongoing, unresolved disagreement between care-giving adults creates confusion for the child (and perhaps for the adults as well). It also undermines a child's emotional sense of safety and parental authority. Testing or pushing limits is the normal developmental "job" of any child. Firm, clear, appropriate parental limit-setting helps children to learn about social values, boundaries, consequences, self-control and the limits of his power. When there are unclear, shifting, or inconsistent limits, both testing behaviors and parent-child conflict may increase and children may learn to play one parent against the other, increasing dissension in the family.

Learning, and practicing, a variety of parenting strategies is helpful. Consistency, predictability and establishing routines are the fundamentals. How you determine, use, and enforce rules are critical. Work toward gradual improvement in your parenting. Knowing and expecting that there will be setbacks can help you to be less disheartened when setbacks inevitably happen. It may seem that nothing works for any period of time, and you may be right. Often ADHD children respond well to novelty. Your child may lose interest in a program that worked well at first. Focusing attention on poor behaviour can wear parents out and exhaust all their behaviour management strategies, leaving them relying heavily on (or only on) punishment. It is difficult to look for and pay attention to positive behaviour when your child seems to be continually misbehaving. ADHD children respond better to encouragement than to criticism, and may have particular difficulty processing verbal commands given impatiently or in anger. Be aware that at times, physical and emotional exhaustion (yours and your child's) is to be expected, and it is important to have a plan. Focus on what both you and your child can learn from conflict and disappointment. Being proactive by having a plan can help to keep you from being thrown off balance as a parent. It is important to find the right strategy, unique to your child, to encourage and ensure his success. Some helpful strategies are: establishing a predictable daily routine, giving short and simple effective commands, with one request at a time, getting visual attention, setting smaller tasks, planing ahead, anticipating boredom, providing structure, using transitional warnings, reducing stimulation when necessary, ignoring minor behaviors such as fidgeting, increasing feedback and immediacy of feedback/consequences.

Be curious, pay attention to what your child's behaviour, challenges and struggles can teach you, and how it can guide your understanding. You can assure yourself that no one knows your child better that you do, and be confident in the decisions and actions you make about his best interests. Both knowing that you are not to blame, and avoiding the blaming others, is helpful. An attitude that both emphasize positives and strengths, and celebrate gains will build self-esteem. Having the belief that your child is adaptable and has great potential will have an impact on all family members.

You may find these strategies hard to implement, especially in the heat of a conflict. Skill development, for you and your child, may be worthwhile. Family therapy, parenting groups, skill development workshops, parent support groups and self-help reading are some strategies that you may find

114 Attention Deficit-Hyperactivity Disorder

helpful. If you have tried something in the past, and it was not helpful, do not be afraid to try it again. Chances are, with an open mind, you may get a different outcome. After all, you and your child have changed somewhat over time, and you may now have a different perspective of the experience.

Self Care

Remember that learning how to care for yourself is especially helpful. Stress is a fact of our lives; it can be helpful to learn how to deal with stress positively and to learn more about self-care. Strive to keep a balance in your life. If you are finding that you are over-involved in any one aspect of your life for too long, whether it is work, sports or hobbies, check out whether you may be trying to escape the problems. Humor, pleasure, joy, laughter, (especially belly laughs), enjoyment of the small daily pleasures of life, sports, interests and hobbies can nourish you emotionally and spiritually. Spending fun time with family and friends can be a great stress reducer. Try to seek support from the community at large, through recreation, volunteering, connecting with other parents who are having similar struggles, etc. Have your world affirmed. Be kind to yourself and your child. Chances are, your goals are not too dissimilar to that of most parents. You want to guide your child in developing the building blocks of "a good life." Foster in him sound judgment, good interpersonal skills, sufficient self-discipline to achieve his dreams and have the chance to make the world a better place, and enough self esteem to care for himself and the world around him. Keep those goals in mind, as the path for both of you continues to unfold. All your hard work has a deep meaning; you are building a parent-child relationship that will last a lifetime. Allow yourself and your child to enjoy each other. Believe in yourself and your child, in your potential to survive, to cope well, to learn, to grow and to thrive.

Sport commentators tell about the athletes who have "heart." These are the persons who may not necessarily be the most talented individuals, but when the chips are down, are able to dig down deep inside themselves to discover reserves that perhaps nobody even suspected were there, least of all themselves. If your family is your most important team, know that you and your child have "heart" and when adversity is all around, it is possible to dig down deep to find strength and resources that will not only get you through, but may even, over time, be transforming. We are all rooting for you!

Other Approaches to Management of ADHD

Men willingly believe what they wish.

Julius Caesar, 100-44 BC

Food sensitivity

In the 1970s, the protest movement against "medicating" school children was still quite loud and strong. During the same period, the "back-to-nature" movement was also gaining momentum. The time was right for the introduction of a different approach to the management of ADHD, which, despite the effectiveness of stimulant therapy, remained a major challenge to all professionals. Dr. Ben Feingold of San Francisco, impressed by the successful treatment of aspirin-sensitive adults with a diet which was free of naturally occurring salicylate (aspirin or ASA is acetylsalicylic acid), hypothesized that hyperactive and learning-disabled children might also respond to this treatment.

Clinical experience had shown that tartrazine, a yellow food coloring, and aspirin could induce identical clinical problems in aspirin-sensitive individuals, even though the two substances are not chemically or structurally related. In some patients, the exclusion of foods containing naturally occurring salicylates did not improve their clinical picture but when tartrazine was also excluded, it did. However, some patients continued to have problems, even on a diet free of salicylates and tartrazine. Dr. Feingold then hypothesized that, since literally thousands of food colorings, flavorings and preservatives are added to our foods during processing, some of them, though not related chemically to aspirin or tartrazine, might be responsible for the clinical picture of aspirin sensitivity. This was the basis for the introduction of Dr. Feingold's K-P diet (named after Kaiser-Permanente Medical Center where Dr. Feingold worked). This diet was salicylate and additive free. He claimed that a number of conditions involving many body organs and systems were manifestations of adverse reactions to some naturally occurring substances in food and/or food additives. He further hypothesized that these adverse reactions occur only in certain genetically predisposed, sensitive individuals.

To this point, a few well-designed studies have demonstrated that some ADHD children show a modest improvement in their behaviour following dietary modifications and that this improvement does not appear to be a placebo effect. Unfortunately, no one can predict which child may benefit from dietary modifications. In practice, the experience of most professionals and families has been that the benefits of changing a child's diet in comparison to other forms of treatment are negligible, or so small, that the inconvenience and expense of the new diet does not warrant a change. Since it is difficult to give a restrictive diet of this nature only to one member of the family, the diet of the entire family has to be changed and this may cause considerable cost, inconvenience and resentment on the part of others in the family.

Since additive-free diets have not been associated with any harmful effects, there is no reason to discourage families who wish to pursue such a diet. Diets which are free of naturally occurring salicylates, however, are restrictive and can result in nutritional deficiencies if they are not under the supervision of a trained dietician. It is imperative that parents consult their family physicians or pediatricians before embarking on this type of diet.

It must be emphasized that the K-P diet is about the removal from the diet of substances to which some people may be sensitive. It is not about the relationship between diet in general and human behaviour. There is lots of evidence that behaviour can be adversely affected in some people by their diet. This will be further discussed below.

Dietary "Deficiencies"

There are a number of studies, which show that increasing certain normal dietary components, which are the precursors (building blocks) of neurotransmitters, increases their concentration in the brain. Likewise there are studies indicating that essential fatty acids, omega 3 and omega 6 and their derivatives, are important for the normal brain functioning through modulating the metabolism and action of certain neurotransmitters. These are interesting and promising new fields of research that will have significant bearing on our understanding of the relationship between food and human behaviour.

There are some individuals who, in order to function normally, require greater amounts of certain micronutrients than required by most people. There is a relatively large body of evidence in the literature that indicates that some people with mood disorders respond better to antidepressant therapy when larger than recommended amounts of one or more micronutrients (vitamins and minerals) are added to their treatment regimen. These individuals have a genetic deficit that interferes either with the absorption or the metabolism of micronutrients. Although supplementing the medical treatment of ADHD children or adults with these micronutrients has not been systematically researched, it is possible that some ADHD individuals might benefit from such supplements. This is particularly the case with the significant number of ADHD children who have coexisting mood and or behaviour disorders (see chapter 11). It is clear that much research in this important field is required. In the meantime, it is prudent to assure that ADHD children receive at least a well balanced diet.

Sugar and ADHD

Many parents claim dramatic improvements in their children's behaviour when their sugar intake is restricted. Blind studies carried out on the effect of sugar on children's behaviour have demonstrated only a placebo effect. In other words, when the parents are blind to the experiment, i.e., they don't know whether the child is receiving sugar or an artificial sweetener in his food or drink), their rating of the child's behaviour does not correspond to what the child is actually taking. This may indicate that the parents are not actually observing the effect of sugar on their children's behaviour. They are, rather, seeing the effect of coloring and flavoring added to candies and other sweets and beverages consumed by their children. Once again, since sugar is not an essential component of human diet, we can not discourage parents who wish to pursue a low sugar diet for their children from doing so.

Caffeine

Recent functional imaging studies of the brains of normal individuals have demonstrated that following ingestion of caffeine there is increased activity in those areas of the brain responsible for focused attention. Caffeine is, of course, the most widely used stimulant in the world. (It is present in coffee and tea and added to many soft drinks.) The amount of caffeine consumed by average individuals has likely no therapeutic effect if the person has ADHD. Much higher doses of caffeine may have some effect in improving attention in ADHD children but would likely have undesirable side effects such as insomnia and rapid heart rates.

Biofeedback

Biofeedback is used principally as a stress reduction technique to teach people to modify certain body responses such as heart rate and muscle tension by controlling and modifying their own electromyogram (EMG). It has been used for both adults and older children to modify their behaviour. Its effectiveness for improving attentive behaviour has not been established.

Brainwave biofeedback attempts to teach people to control their behaviour through controlling their brainwave patterns using Electroencephalogram (EEG).

EEG biofeedback is considered experimental and not widely available.

It must be emphasized that when a child is given any form of treatment, whether it be stimulant therapy, K-P diet, low sugar diet or other forms of therapy, the benefits and potential harmful side-effects for the child and his family must be carefully considered. Some form of treatment may harm the child by depriving him of a more effective means of treatment. Other forms of treatment may create a great deal of family stress. This may be the case when, for the benefit of the affected child, the

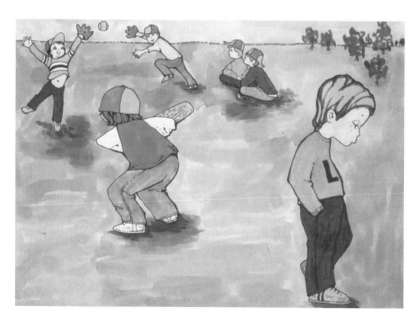

entire family is placed on a diet, which may be costly, inconvenient or unpalatable to the entire family.

11   ADHD Complications

Samuel Y-Y Chang, MD

No excellent soul is exempt from a mixture of madness.

Aristotle, 384-322 BC

It is reported that about four fifth of ADHD children show evidence of the presence of other developmental or behavioral problems (American Psychiatric Association, DSM IV). Children with these associated problems have complex or complicated ADHD and those without them have simple ADHD. In medical terminology we call these associated problems *comorbidities*, meaning conditions coexisting with ADHD. They may be present from early infancy. These include mental retardation, visual and or auditory perceptual problems associated with learning disabilities and signs of autistic spectrum.

However, other associated problems (behavioral, mood and thinking problems) may develop in untreated or inadequately treated individuals with ADHD. They are expressions of the same underlying brain problem. Like in any other medical condition, the earlier the diagnosis of ADHD is made and treatment begun, the less the risk of developing these complications. An individual with untreated or inadequately treated ADHD can, over time, show deterioration in other related areas of brain function, just as an individual with poorly controlled diabetes can develop cardiovascular problems or other complications of diabetes.

Of course, ADHD can also lead to other conditions such as orthopedic injuries of impulsive children, motor vehicle accidents in inattentive and impulsive adolescents and numerous mental, emotional and social problems stemming from substance abuse in poorly treated or untreated ADHD in childhood.

How do Complications Arise?

a) No treatment

The most severe complications are the result of the lack of diagnosis of ADHD that may lead to the full forces of untreated ADHD being unleashed on the child and his family members. The child may be seen as bad or unmanageable and the parents may be seen as incompetent even though they have successfully raised other well-behaved children. The parents may also blame themselves for the child's misbehaviors. These conscious and often unconscious dynamics then set up the child and the family for unhealthy interactions and functioning. The end result can be quite severe behavioral problems, to the point that crimes may be committed and the child's life course altered.

The negative life events to which an undiagnosed ADHD child is exposed, such as academic failure, poor social interactions, isolation from peers and troubled authority relationships at home and school, can lead to behavioral and emotional complications. The most common of these are anxiety disorders and mood disorders.

One of the most debilitating and chronic conditions that can result from untreated ADHD is **substance abuse** (alcohol and street drugs) and its consequences. A recent compilation of many studies comparing treated versus untreated ADHD patients revealed that the risk of substance abuse doubles in untreated ADHD individuals over a lifetime, but is about six times greater in adolescence.. Since the human brain continues to mature until late teens and early twenties, it is clear to see the devastating effects that substance abuse and substance-abusing culture can have on *personality formation*, which is the main developmental task of adolescence. **Personality** is the technical term for how we perceive and interpret the world and human interactions and respond to them. If we perceive these as hostile and persecuting, we respond in an angry, paranoid, guarded or withdrawn manner. The development of a *personality disorder* is perhaps the ultimate complication of untreated ADHD since it is regarded as essentially permanent and not really treatable. It can only be modified at best.

b) Inadequate treatment

Recent scientific endeavors have proven the superiority of combined optimal medication and behavioral therapies to either only medication or only behavioral therapies. We now know that optimal treatment with *remission* as its goal is not only desirable but also achievable. **Remission** means that that the treated individual is indistinguishable from others of the same developmental level. The concept of remission has been a significant progress in ADHD treatment. We are no longer content with, nor have as our goal, improvement of behaviour, but complete normalization. The complications of inadequate or suboptimal treatment are higher than optimal treatment. The optimal treatment of ADHD means looking for complications, i.e., comorbidities and treating them at the same time.

c) Genetic factors

There are times when despite expert diagnosis, optimal treatment and thorough follow-up by an expert team of professionals, maximum patient compliance and unwavering parental and family support, outcomes of treatment are still suboptimal. This does not mean that anyone is to be blamed. Rather, it would mean that one's genetic endowment might make even the best treatment suboptimal. Examples of this are the person with profound sensitivities to medication that prevents optimal dosage or lack of response to the most expert dosage, or timing of medication or even the combination of medications. We know that many of these effects are heritable and scientists are working to find solutions for them (see chapter 4, causes of ADHD, possible role of nutritional factors).

While we are waiting for these solutions it is good to remember that we are talking about the risk and not the certainties of developing complications. In other words, even the worst outcomes of treatment do not necessarily lead to disaster. Many well-known historical personalities suffered from ADHD and never received treatment for it!

Common Comorbidities/Complications

a) Mood disorders

These are estimated to be present in about one quarter of patient with ADHD and include:

- **Chronic low grade depression**.

- **Major depression**, i.e., high-grade depression that may be chronic or transient.

- **Bipolar disorder**, i.e., cycling mood disorders with both lows (depression) and ups (elation and/or irritability) often in very quick swinging "mixed states" in children.

- **Seasonal affective disorder**, i.e., seasonal fluctuations of mood when short daylight hours result in depression. It responds to light therapy but is harder to diagnose in school children as short daylight months are times of peak school stress as well.

b) Anxiety disorders

These are estimated to present in about one third of patients with ADHD and include:

- **Generalized anxiety disorder** affecting many areas of one's life and interferes with functioning.

- **Simple phobias** such as fear of heights or public speaking.

- **Panic disorder**, i.e., unprovoked and unpredictable episode of panic attacks that can be disabling.

- **Obsessive-compulsive disorder**, i.e., use of repetitive thoughts (obsessions) and/or repetitive actions/ rituals (compulsions) to cope with anxiety provoking situations; for example excessive fear of having done something wrong or fear of germs and excessive hand washing.

c) Behavioural problems/substance abuse

Behavioral problems are some of the most common complications of ADHD and increase the risk of substance abuse.

- **Oppositional–defiant disorder** starts typically in childhood with both passive opposition to the rules and active defiance.

- **Conduct disorder.** The child or adolescent consistently impinges on the right of others and may engage in criminal activities. This introduction to the legal/justice system often leads to more negative peer group affiliation (gangs, criminals) and to adoption of these behaviors to deal with the world as an adult with *"antisocial personality disorder."*

Added to these behaviors is the increased risk of substance abuse in untreated ADHD children. There is no evidence of increased substance abuse in treated ADHD children. In fact, there is a two-fold decrease of risk with medication therapy, including stimulant therapy.

As mentioned earlier in this chapter, substance abuse in adolescents is associated with the risk of insult to their still maturing brains with the resulting maladaptive response to the world that they perceive as hostile, and to the development of personality disorders.

d) Tic disorder

Tics are involuntary vocal or motor movements and are often genetically linked to ADHD They may occur concurrently with ADHD, whether on or off medication. However, stiumulant medications can aggravate tics when they appear. If present, they should be treated concurrently with ADHD. Anextreme example of a tic disorder is Tourette's syndrome.

e) Physical injury/ motor vehicle accidents

These are common complications of untreated ADHD resulting from hyperactivity and impulsivity, which can continue into adolescence and adulthood. They can cause much grief to the individuals and their families and significantly increase the cost of health care to society.

f) Others

There are many more individual, familial, social and societal complications of untreated ADHD that has put the disorder into the realm of public health problems. In fact, it has been designated as such by the Center for Disease Control in the United States.

12   Adolescents with ADHD

Geraldine Farrelly, MD

The Wildest colts make the best horses.

Themistocles, 512-499 B.C.

Adolescence is a time of tumultuous change. Surging hormones, increasing peer pressure, search for self-identity and the intensified struggle for independence go hand in hand with tremendous transformations that are taking place physically, intellectually, emotionally and socially. It is both a terrifying and exciting time for these young people who must go through difficult transition times and the adjustment to junior high school from elementary school.

The ADHD adolescents, either diagnosed or undiagnosed, have even more challenges to face in the junior high school environment as they often struggle to cope with extra responsibilities and increased expectations. They have particular difficulties compensating for their poor organizational skills while attempting to meet the increased demands in these settings. As a result, they often feel overwhelmed and frustrated.

In the previous chapters of this book we discussed ADHD, its causes, complications and treatments primarily to help parents and teachers understand this complex condition. One of the most important goals of this chapter is to ensure that physicians who might read it become familiar with the diversity of the ADHD presentations in the adolescent population and to learn that with proper intervention strategies, the prognosis for these young people is indeed very promising.

How adolescents with ADHD present to the professional vary greatly and quite differently from that of the elementary school children with ADHD. Understanding these differences is essential for a proper assessment and management of ADHD in adolescents.

In the following pages we use the word "teens" to cover individuals 11 to 20 years old.

Finding the Right Professional

Parents seeking help for their teen need to determine if a particular professional is knowledgeable, not only in the area of ADHD, but is also comfortable and empathic in the presence of teenagers. Included in this chapter are some practical tips to help parents find a good fit among their teen, family and professional; an essential step to fostering a successful outcome.

ADHD Characteristics in Adolescents

Core symptoms of ADHD; i.e., inattention with or without hyperactivity/impulsivity, usually persist into adolescence (85%) and adulthood (60-70%). While some symptoms such as hyperactivity diminish, others, such as organizational difficulties, become more obvious. ADHD can therefore manifest differently at different ages and stages of development, and as a result, the diagnosis can be missed or overlooked if parents or professionals are not aware of these varied presentations.

Hallmarks of ADHD in Teens

Hyperactivity maybe replaced in many by internal feelings of restlessness or more obvious fidgetiness, from age 11 years onwards.

Impulsivity can lead to poor choices and risky behaviour impacting the teen, family members, peers and others.

Inattention, distractibility, procrastination, poor listening skills, poor time management, misplacing, losing, forgetting items organizational difficulties (*poor executive function*) are hallmarks of ADHD and may only become obvious for the first time in the pre-teen/teen/young adult years. Many bright and pleasant individuals with ADHD, but without hyperactivity/impulsivity or behavioral problems, have gone undiagnosed for years. Most often, girls fit into this category and are overlooked, but many boys can also belong to this group.

Other Complicating Factors

The emergence of other coexisting disorders (comorbidities) such as anxiety/depression, oppositional defiance or conduct disorders can complicate the picture and need to be addressed and treated. Previously unrecognized learning difficulties or academic underachievement caused by years of undiagnosed or poorly managed ADHD can cause secondary feelings of frustration and loss of self-esteem. These feelings can result in externalizing behaviors, such as acting out and temper outbursts, or internalizing symptoms, such as anxiety, which further complicate the assessment and diagnosis.

Diagnostic Differences

The diagnostic process, although similar to that for the elementary school child, is more complex for the adolescent and takes a significantly longer time. Parents must have patience and be prepared for a lengthy assessment. A careful and accurate evaluation is far superior to a rushed, possibly inaccurate, diagnosis. Other conditions that can mimic ADHD need to be carefully considered or excluded. Coexisting problems can emerge more often in adolescence, but may not be obvious. In some cases these co-occurring conditions may overshadow the diagnosis of ADHD. It is therefore imperative that the clinician conducts a thorough investigation. The history, supplemented with questionnaires from other observers, is the key to diagnosis. Using good detective skills, inclusive and exclusive criteria from DSM IV can be identified in order to conclude whether ADHD is the sole diagnosis or other diagnoses coexist. Once the diagnosis has been established, a proper management plan can be outlined.

Management Strategies for Adolescents with Comorbitities

As with elementary school children who may have comorbidities, it is usually best to treat the ADHD first unless the co-occurring condition is extremely severe and demands priority in treatment (for example, severe clinical depression). Often a coexisting condition, such as anxiety, improves once the ADHD is under control. Other times, the coexisting conditions may require treatment at the same time. Once ADHD is under better control, it is easier to determine if the individual will benefit from other interventions which may have been difficult before (for example, counselling for depression, anxiety, other medications, etc.).

Practical Pointers for Parents and Professionals

Don't Judge a Book by its Cover

Many professionals feel intimidated by teens. Their attitude and attire sometimes can be outrageous – from hostile to friendly, happy to sad, insightful to spiteful, jock to Spock, nerdy to preppy or pleasant to pouty much to their parents' dismay. However, looks and attitude can be very deceiving indeed. Unfortunately, judgments and labels are attached to this population who may actually be just very normal teens struggling for recognition, acceptance and attention. ADHD teens, as a group, are no more different in this respect from their non-ADHD counterparts but may take things to the extreme.

Put Prejudice in its Place

Like the iceberg, what lies beneath is worth exploring, acknowledging and helping. ADHD teens are often shy individuals with poor self-esteem, struggling for acceptance in any group; some put on an act of bravado for maximum attention to cover up inadequacies in school and elsewhere while others are already sliding the slippery slop to troubled pathways and negative peer influence. It is important for professionals and parents to put their prejudices aside and not judge these youngsters too harshly or quickly.

Establish Rapport

When this most vulnerable population enters a professional's office, the opportunity for a vital connection can be established or lost depending on the ability and flexibility of the professional to look past appearance. The same is true for the parent who struggles with their child's image and ignores the real issues.

Innocent Until Proven Guilty

It is important to remember that individuals with ADHD have often been misjudged and their actions misinterpreted. As a result they may have been subject to punishment, embarrassment, humiliation and rejection in many situations. They may arrive at the professional's office under duress feeling misunderstood and miserable, expecting yet another condemnation. It is imperative for parents and professionals to keep an open mind even if the evidence presented by school or others seems damning.

Listen to Their Story

Their version of events (i.e., what led to a suspension or other scenario) must be heard. Listen to the whole story. It is crucial to understand that gentle probing, rather than angry accusations help unravel all the important clues and a clearer picture emerges. Once they feel they are being listened to with respect and not being judged unfairly, they are likely willing to go through with the assessment and also much more likely to adhere to the recommendations. Once a therapeutic alliance is formed the stage is set for an excellent future relationship.

Divide and Conquer

At times, when an unwilling teen is dragged to the professional's office, not quite kicking and screaming but decidedly against their wishes, a tense atmosphere can ensue. This, coupled with the fact that the parents and their teen are also in conflict, can seriously jeopardize the interview. It is best to diffuse this uncomfortable situation by acting as a mediator, laying out the ground rules for a successful interview from the onset. Conduct separate interviews for teens and parents as well as joint interviews. This allows each party to speak more freely, enhancing communication and negotiation.

Negotiate not Negate

Having a professional listen to both parents and teen with empathy can often result in more willingness to compromise on both sides. After discussing the issues and negotiating, some household rules are deemed essential; others are changed or modified to each other's mutual satisfaction. This validates each party's concern and allows for a sense of accomplishment.

Poor Time Concept

Morning routines are often a challenge even for the well-meaning, well-behaved ADHD individual and their families. They require constant reminders to stay on task, follow directions and be aware of time constraints. Those with a combination of a difficult temperament and/or hyperactive/impulsive behaviour can place extra demands on all involved. These challenges often result in feelings of anger, frustration and stress for all family members. Getting these individuals out the door on time with all their necessary belongings can be quite an achievement.

Transitions

Once the supports of elementary school are no longer present, difficulties with transition to junior high school may occur. Adolescents with ADHD often grapple with their organizational difficulties. This change of school system with multiple teachers, different expectations, increased responsibility and independence, deadlines to meet and lockers to manage can overwhelm, resulting in plummeting grades and frustration. Similarly, young adult/college/university students who leave the structure and support of living at home behind to embark on a college or university career can face the same problems. Once the scaffolding is removed, things can start falling apart, reflecting in poor grades and this may be a significant clue that there may be underlying attentional issues which need to be explored.

Read Between the Lines

Reviewing old report cards, grade by grade, will give valuable clues to helping unravel the diagnosis at a later age. Often, it is what is not said but what is implied that gives weight to suspicions that these "new characteristics" were in fact evident in earlier years but were unrecognized as such. Key comments such as "Improved focus this term," "starting to complete assignments better," usually appear on term three and four report cards when they were never mentioned as being a problem prior to that. Teachers try to be as positive as possible writing report cards. Parents may realize they have been spending inordinate amounts of time helping with homework and organization over the years in order to keep up with assignments and grades. However, this may not be obvious to the teachers. The teen or young adult may admit to struggling to focus in class, or deny that it is a problem confusing boredom with daydreaming, and inattention with lack of motivation.

The Consistently Inconsistent Report Card

It is important to be aware that report cards that are classic for the ADHD individuals show marks that are not only inconsistent from subject to subject (i.e., 80% to 30% etc.) but within the subject themselves. When scrutinizing their report cards, it is not uncommon to discover marks ranging from 100% in some quizzes to 0% for not handing in assignments, to 80% in assignments completed and handed in, to 50% in some tests, etc. Their marks and the teacher comments are all over the map. These inconsistencies are consistent with classic characteristics of ADHD. This pattern of performance should always be explored when considering the possibility of an underlying ADHD, particularly in post-elementary teens.

Simple Strategies to the Rescue

Establish contact with at least one teacher who can make contact with the others and set up a system to coordinate improved communication between school, the ADHD individual and parents (i.e., agenda charts, monthly calendars, homework times, study skills and organizational classes, email, etc.). Therefore, at least everyone is aware of assignments that need to be done, when they are due, and what tests are planned. This will ensure that more timely intervention can occur.

Get it in Writing

A visit to the professional for assessment of ADHD can be overwhelming for the family. There can be information overload with lots of suggestions given or too little information given. The professionals should give parents written instructions, such as handouts, or parents should write down this information and keep a file on their child/teen. This ensures better follow through and more effective communication with other agencies and solid references for future meetings.

It's a Family Affair

It is important for the professional and parent to remember that ADHD is a strongly inherited condition. Therefore the likelihood of the parent in question having similar traits (i.e., losing, forgetting, being late, lacking routine, etc.) is quite high and should be kept in mind when dealing with management issues at home and school.

Peer Differences

In many instances, ADHD individuals struggle to keep up with their peers and not just inside the classroom. Their inability to listen attentively to conversations, their tendency to go off topic, miss the directions in sports, forget to bring the necessary item/equipment for outings or sports (working memory) and turn up late for events often makes them the last ones picked for group activities. The active, boisterous, impulsive types are avoided or tormented.

These traits are an added burden for any teenager struggling to fit in and be part of the crowd. It erodes their self-esteem little by little. Unfortunately, some become involved with less desirable peer groups, leading to risky and troubling behaviors both in and out of school.

Other factor that may also make many ADHD teens stand apart from their peers is their apparent lack of maturity and insight. Many have not developed an interest in the more sophisticated hobbies of their peers (fashion, opposite sex, music, etc.). Instead, they may still prefer to play with Lego, Barbies, etc. and enjoy the company of younger children. Unfortunately, this may lead to teasing or ridicule when exposed to their peer group.

Good Friends

ADHD individuals who are very charismatic, with excellent social skills and creativity are fun to be with. They often have a posse of friends willing to organize them to ensure their presence at whatever social or sporting event they are expected to attend (e.g., phoning them early in the morning, picking them up, making sure they have the necessary equipment for a ski trip, etc.). These compensatory strategies, although helpful, may mask the underlying organization and attention difficulties but salvage self-esteem.

Gender Differences

Over the years, ADHD has been diagnosed significantly more frequently in males. Recent changes to the Diagnostic Criteria for ADHD, with the introduction of DSM IV in 1994, have helped uncover many more females with ADHD. Many of these females met the criteria for predominantly inattentive ADHD and in the past were often overlooked. Girls with ADHD, combined type, stand out from their peers. Although most are recognized as having ADHD in elementary school and treated appropriately, others are missed.

Prior to teen years, girls in general have a tendency to want to please, fit in socially, achieve academically and not cause trouble at school or home. Some may appear shy and "daydreamy" while others can be bossy and intrusive. Excessive talking can be a hallmark of ADHD in females, as opposed to the physical hyperactivity seen in their male counterparts. Comments on report cards may indicate this and thus it is important that the professional involved and the parent recognize this as a possible indicator of ADHD in combination with other characteristics.

Anxiety traits can be present and should be explored and addressed. Girls often internalize their frustrations and fears and sometimes complaints such as headaches and abdominal pains may appear. In junior high school and into higher grades, girls, in their quest to strive for academic accomplishments, may have a tendency to be very hard on themselves. Many spend hours working on written projects in an effort to complete them within the deadlines given. Their poor organizational skills and time management skills force them to spend these unnecessary hours that others with similar intellect without ADHD can accomplish much faster. Although they may be keeping up on the surface, the cost is often too much, leaving them little or no time for recreation. Their irritability may only be apparent in the home when, finally, they may take out their frustrations on family members. Hormonal changes and the presence of premenstrual syndrome (PMS) may also contribute to their changing emotions during these crucial and formative years. This may influence medication management of their ADHD. In some, risky behaviors may escalate resulting in breaking curfews, non-adherence to rules, poor choice of peers, unsafe sex, pregnancy, sexually transmitted diseases, experimentation with alcohol, drugs and cigarettes and eventually leaving home and school. All of these issues can come as a complete surprise for parents when their daughters reach their teen years, as many of these individuals had been compliant, respectful and motivated in younger years. Again, this stresses the need for early recognition and treatment of ADHD in order to prevent additional problems in teen years for those at risk.

In adulthood, many females with ADHD, when faced with the added responsibilities of having to care for their children and husband, run a household and work outside the home, may find it very difficult to cope. The extra demands on their poor organizational and time management skills plus the fact that they often have children with ADHD, can result in an unstructured home life, with many missed or late appointments and deadlines and a great deal of frustration. Others find a partner who is very organized and survive. Research is ongoing on possible gender differences in ADHD that may prove very helpful for its diagnosis and management.

Preserve Self-esteem

It is crucial to emphasize individual strengths in ADHD individuals in order to promote their self-esteem and success. Unfortunately, by the time they reach the teen years, many have equated lack of production at school with not "being smart." They need to be reassured and helped to "show case" their talents which may previously have been overlooked. Many, when ADHD has been fully identified and treated, are able to focus enough to be successful in various situations both inside and outside of the classroom (e.g., written production, art, sports, music, etc.). These accomplishments allow them to finally dream of future careers and lifestyles previously thought to be unattainable.

The Good News

Many of the characteristics of ADHD, which seem to be a drawback in the earlier years of life, can be turned around and used to an advantage later in life. We should, therefore, remain optimistic about future outcomes, particularly in the identified and well-managed ADHD individuals. Some ADHD characteristics can be assets, not hindrances. The passion, enthusiasm, creativity, tenacity, determination and high energy levels often seen in some ADHD individuals, when focused on an area of special interest for them, can be very successfully transferred to careers of their choice. Parents and professionals are urged to promote these positive assets when dealing with ADHD individuals, particularly those who are struggling and frustrated, in order to encourage their continued motivation for success.

The Holistic Approach

Teens are notorious for skipping breakfast in order to enjoy the luxury of sleeping an extra 5or 10 minutes in the morning. Often, they also miss lunch or just grab junk food and pop in order to be with their peers. It is important for parents, teens and professionals to work out a strategy, including night time and morning routines, to ensure there is time for a proper breakfast every morning, particularly when their appetite at lunchtime may be depressed due to their medications. The importance of good nutrition for proper growth, as well as for enhanced ability to focus and physical activity, should be stressed.

Many teens spend an enormous amount of time playing video/computer games or chat online or on the phone. They watch too much TV instead of being involved in recreational activities such as sports, arts or drama classes etc. They should be strongly encouraged to take up some form of physical exercise and other activities to promote a healthy life style. Physical exercise helps to decrease stress and frustration, promotes self-esteem and enhances the ability to focus. By writing these recommendations on a prescription pad, the physician can deliver the message that these instructions are important and need to be followed just like those for medications.

Medication in Adolescence — The Evidence

Although there has been overwhelming validation for the use of psycho-stimulant medications (Ritalin, Dexedrine,

Concerta, Aderall XR) and the new non-stimulant medication (Strattera) as first line treatment for ADHD, it is still advisable to approach the subject of medication with caution. Many families prefer to try other strategies prior to using medication or they are apprehensive regarding medication and, therefore, need time to reflect and adjust to this possibility by educating themselves and their teens. It is unwise to prescribe medication at the time of the initial visit. However, it is very appropriate to discuss medication if the situation demands more immediate intervention or at a later date when the family wishes to pursue this treatment. Each situation is unique depending on circumstances; i.e., the severity of impairments, the threat of expulsion from school, etc. It is important to know that unless the teenager is in full agreement with the discussion to try medication, the outcome may be doomed to failure.

Use Long Acting Medication

The use of long acting medication is preferable for most ADHD individuals at any age, but it is essential for adolescents with ADHD. Adolescents are more prone to non-compliance than elementary school children for a variety of reasons. For example lunchtime is no longer routine and there is lack of supervision so a lunchtime dose of medication may be missed. Peer pressure can be higher and the quest for independence and not wanting to be controlled, as well as the desire to fit in and not appear different or embarrassed at all costs, may lead to "forgetfulness" and non-compliance. Of course, forgetfulness can also be genuine which, understandably, could cause them not to take, or misplace, their medication.

The newer, long-acting medications, Adderall XR and Concerta, allow for 10 – 12 plus hours of coverage and Strattera works for about 24 hours. However, health care benefits in many provinces in Canada will not cover the costs of these newer and improved formulations, thereby limiting the choices for some individuals. In those cases, Dexedrine Spansules would be the most acceptable alternative. Please refer to the chapter on medication for more details regarding medications used for treatment of ADHD.

Whatever the choice of medication, the teen must be an integral part of the team evaluating the medication trial. This is the only way to ensure a successful outcome. A combination of medication and strategies to use at home and school promotes better follow-through for the long term.

Many myths abound regarding medication use and these should be discussed with the family and dispelled. Parents also have concerns regarding possible long-term growth problems, drug dependency, sleep problems, etc. In my practice, after following young children on medication (some for almost 20 years), the majority have grown into tall adults depending on family genetics (males range 5'7" to 6'7"). Some did not start going through their growth spurts until grade 10 or 11 and started to grow tall in their late teens and early twenties, just like their fathers and grandfathers before them. While some may have had a decreased appetite at lunchtime and sleep issues, others were able to eat better and sleep better due to their increased ability to focus on the task at hand (lunch, dinner) and bedtime routine. Having a better day in general seems to improve the ability to settle down to sleep. None had developed problems with high blood pressure or cardiac problems at the time of discharge after many years of follow up. The literature indicates that ADHD individuals who are well treated and optimally managed are significantly less likely to have problems with drug addictions in later life and that coincides with my personal observations over the years. Although these observations are limited to a clinical setting and not long-term research, it is certainly encouraging and reassuring to see firsthand that a significant number of treated ADHD individuals over the long-term are indeed healthy and functioning well in life. It is always important to remember that medication is only part of an overall management plan.

ADHD Teens – Triumph over Adversity

This chapter is dedicated to the hundreds of individuals with ADHD who allowed me to share their very intimate personal journeys through childhood, adolescence and adulthood over a 20-plus year period. What they have taught me goes far beyond the confines of academic textbooks and research papers. Their shared experiences, their struggles and triumphs, have shaped my knowledge, clinical skills and teaching skills in the area of ADHD. To them, I owe a great deal of personal and professional gratification and I thank all of them.

Sharing some stories of times spent with these most interesting and mostly likeable people during my long years of practice will hopefully help parents, individuals with ADHD and professionals to feel encouraged and empowered to go forward with a more positive outlook for the future.

The long-term consequences of untreated or poorly managed ADHD are well-known and well-documented in the literature and elsewhere in this book. However, in this chapter, on a more positive note, I would like to focus on the successful outcomes. Often these success stories of triumph over adversity are overlooked and buried under the doom and gloom of the sad outcomes.

Their Stories . . .

The Energetic Engineer

I was first introduced to this delightful, active five-year-old in ECS and confirmed a diagnosis of ADHD combined type. With a combination of medication, and home and school support he became an excellent student and a valuable team player in hockey and football. There were occasional disruptions in his progress along the way, mainly coinciding with transitions at school and home, adolescence, missed medication or need for medication readjustment. However, he graduated with honors from high school, received a diploma from Southern Alberta Institute of Technology (SAIT), a unique new two-year program, and graduated from University of Calgary with a degree in Engineering.

I was privileged to follow him every few months from five years of age through to his Engineering degree completion, at first accompanied by his mother and in later years alone. I watched him grow into a tall, 6'.2", muscular, academically achieving, happy, socially well-adjusted young man who was also an accomplished athlete. I looked forward to our meetings and enjoyed our conversations. Reviewing college and university report cards was indeed a pleasure. Although he continued to require his medication (Dexedrine Long Acting Spansules) in order to focus, control impulses and remain organized both in class, in the workforce and in sports, the dosage of his medication significantly decreased through college and university years. It was very encouraging to see his successful transformation to young adulthood over the years. I know that he is a valuable member of society and an excellent role model.

Lessons Learned

The bright hyperactive/impulsive child, without other coexisting diagnoses and with a good home and school support, optimum medication management and frequent follow-up, can achieve an excellent outcome in life. The ability and opportunity to turn negative traits such as hyperactivity/ impulsivity into a goal-directed high energy in a career of one's choice and on the football field is indeed the perfect way to compensate and achieve.

- Medication dosage can be significantly reduced in late teen/young adulthood for those who still require medication.

- Long-acting medication gives superior control over ADHD symptoms especially in teens/adults.

- It's very rewarding for professionals to follow teens and young adults and witness their successes in life.

Chef Charming

This future chef was in grade 2 when we met and diagnosed ADHD. Thankfully, an astute psychologist during a cognitive (I.Q.) testing noted symptoms of this disorder and recommended a referral to determine if the child met the criteria for diagnosis of ADHD.

This young man had a very difficult time throughout his elementary years and early junior high, mainly because he was bullied and belittled by his peers. He presented as an awkward looking boy whose glasses, unfortunately, were hugely magnified and made him stand out from his peers who took every opportunity to taunt and intimidate him. His chronically ill, impoverished single mother tried her best to protect him with little support from the school. Poor self-esteem, lack of social acceptance, lack of athletic accomplishments and academic underachievement were all major issues during those turbulent times. Medication helped enormously with his focus, but strategies for success were limited in his school environments.

Finally, a fresh start at a new supportive high school, in combination with optimal medication use, home support and a physical transformation. changed his life for the better. He exchanged his unflattering glasses for contact lenses; he adopted a more trendy approach to dressing and hair style, grew tall and confident and at last he achieved academic and social success.

Following his progress into the prestigious SAIT professional chef program with exemplary marks was indeed a privilege. His social life soared and he graduated with his red SEAL in Culinary Arts and a diploma. His visits were out of the ordinary as I had the great pleasure of inspecting and learning about his culinary tools and receiving great culinary tips.

Lessons learned

- Ritalin S.R. (Long-acting Ritalin) can work for the chosen few (with a less than 30% success rate in most and only a duration of action of 4 – 6 hours in many- luckily for this boy lasted 8 hours).

- In the late afternoon he did require Ritalin Short-acting medication for extended coverage. Dexedrine Spansules (Long-acting) did not work for him. The newest 12-hour and 24-hour medications were not yet formulated or available at that time.

- As the Fairytale goes the "frog" turned into prince charming. In other words, with continued compliance with medications, long-term support and management; a turbulent life can improve dramatically in a highly motivated pleasant ADHD individual.

- Professionals can enjoy conversations with their adolescent/young adults, discussing their shared topics of interest, and learn at the same time.

The CSI Guy

This pleasant, bright boy who had achieved academic success throughout elementary school arrived in my office with plummeting grades on entering junior high (Grade 7, Alberta). Although there had been no obvious problems in elementary school, reviewing old report cards had just some hints of possible focusing issues from time to time. According to his junior high teachers, he had many assignments missing, incomplete or overdue. His poor organizational skills were a concern and he was underachieving academically as a result. He admitted to having problems focusing also and he was diagnosed with ADHD, Predominantly Inattentive Type.

This diagnosis and the fact that this student was having problems in junior high came as a complete surprise to his parents who already had two identified ADHD younger boys in the home. One of the brothers was diagnosed at four and a half years old with severe combined type, the other in grade 3, also with combined type. Both brothers also had significant learning disabilities and some other comorbidities. The father also had a recent diagnosis of ADHD after recognizing similar traits in himself although he had a successful career and family life. Compared to his younger brothers, this older boy had appeared entirely normal to his family.

The mother in this family was an amazingly organized, caring person who provided an excellent supportive, structured and consistent environment for all family members. The combination of being bright and having a happy, secure home life and good elementary school was a plus for him.

Once diagnosed, treated with medication and with continued home support and strategies to improve organization, he excelled through junior high, high school and university obtaining his degree in criminology. Of note was that he, his family and school noticed an immediate improvement in his ability to focus the initial day he started his medication. He remained on medication through his student days with minimal change in dosage (Dexedrine Spansules, 15mg). He grew into a tall, likeable, successful young man and a good football player who also enjoyed a well-rounded social and happy family life.

Like many people who grew up enjoying mystery books and detective shows, forensic science holds a fascination for me. Reviewing this excellent students subject matter and report cards each term allowed me the pleasure of not only monitoring his success and medications but also gave me the opportunity to learn more about forensic facts. His visits were indeed always most enjoyable and fascinating.

Lessons Learned

- Transition from elementary school to junior high can indeed be overwhelming especially with ADHD, diagnosed or undiagnosed.

- The diagnosis of ADHD may be first confirmed in many male and female students only after elementary and secondary school years, when increased demands are placed on their organizational skills (executive function) in environments with less structured supports and overall consistency.

- Appropriate medication at the optimum dosage for a specific individual can seem like a miracle on the first day.

- Big guy, small dosage of medication (Dexedrine Spansule, 15 mg) met this individual's needs. Always make sure to tailor the medication and dosage to fit each person irrespective of their size or age. This young man's other family members required larger dosages and a combination of other medications for their coexisting diagnoses.

- The privilege of being involved in the lives of such remarkable individuals brings untold rewards to parents and professionals alike.

The Pleasant Princess

Several years ago I had the pleasure of meeting the "princess" with ADHD combined type who was referred because of medication management issues. Every medication available at that time had been tried unsuccessfully except for short-acting Ritalin, which had been helpful for focusing. Even then, this was not providing sufficient coverage or working as effectively as in the past. This pretty, polite, petite, bright grade 5 student was successful academically, but she struggled excessively to keep up because of poor organizational skills. This resulted in hours of extra time spent "studying" in order to keep up with the demands of her private school with high expectations for success. Although she was highly motivated to do well, it was impossible for her to focus and sit in one place unless her medication was in effect.

Unfortunately she only received a maximum of 3 hours coverage at a time from her Ritalin. And for some time, her days were like being on a rollercoaster – focused, not focused – and leading to inconsistent performance at school. This presented some challenges for her parents and siblings at home. She was required to take her medication at least four times daily, quite a challenge for a non-ADHD individual, never mind a person with ADHD. Fortunately she was well liked at school and the extent of her difficulties without medication was understood by all. She was reminded in a positive way to take her medication often. Thankfully, she never viewed these reminders in a negative way as she realized how important medication was for her performance both inside and outside the classroom. Her family was exceptionally understanding and provided a caring, supportive, structured environment for her. A psychologist provided organizational strategies and counselling for some anxiety traits. With the onset of adolescence and transitions at school, she was tried again on long-acting medication with no success. Finally, with the arrival of Adderall XR (long-acting dextroamphetamine), she eventually had 8 hours of continuous coverage and the addition of Ritalin in the evening gave her the ability to focus during that time. Concerta (long-acting Ritalin) did not work for this young lady. Currently she is a very successful student in grade 11 at a new high school. With her intelligence, motivation, determination and family support, she should continue to be very successful in her future endeavours.

Lessons Learned

* Having a high IQ does not guarantee success in life.

* A supportive, caring, structured and understanding family is desirable for any child but is essential for the ADHD child.

* Limited organizational skills severely impact the lives of even the brightest and most motivated ADHD individuals especially in junior and senior high schools.

* Although short-acting Ritalin worked for this child, Concerta (long-acting Ritalin) did not.

* Even though Dexedrine Spansules was a failure for her, Adderall XR was a success.

* Always keep trying until the optimum medication is found for each individual.

Spectacular Spectrums

One of the most puzzling cases from the late '80s turned out to have a diagnosis of ADHD, complicated by Asperger syndrome, anxiety and obsessive/compulsive disorder (OCD). His brother also has ADHD combined type, mild Asperger syndrome and anxiety but not OCD.

The reason I'm including these delightful boys in the story section, is that too often children/teens like these boys are misdiagnosed or overlooked. They end up being either inappropriately treated or only treated for one of their diagnoses. Thus, they remain not only misunderstood, but also unable to realize their potential in life.

To this day I still meet preteens and teens who have slipped through the cracks and might only be diagnosed as gifted, or Gifted LD with or without ADHD who, in actual fact, meet the criteria for Asperger's syndrome. On the other hand, children with significant ADHD, predominately inattentive type, have been labelled with Asperger's syndrome. Often their ADHD has gone undetected or untreated, creating a false impression of Asperger's syndrome. Their social difficulties may have been caused by the fact that, due to their inattention, they rarely initiate a conversation or may lose track of the conversation. They may also have fleeting eye contact when spoken to as a result of their distractibility.

Asperger syndrome falls under the umbrella of Autistic Spectrum Disorders. It was described by Hans Asperger in 1944 and it only came to prominence in the mid-80s. Children with this disorder are usually bright, have normal language but may not use language for conversation unless they are talking about topics of specific interest to them or to obtain their wants and needs. The areas of special interest vary from person to person but often relate to trains, cars, machinery, animals, sport scores, etc. Their artwork, reading materials, written stories, movies, drama and conversation usually revolve around these topics. Often they have hypersensitivity to sounds, smells, tastes, touch and feel of certain clothes, etc. Consequently exposure to certain items in the environments can trigger monumental overreactions and huge meltdowns. They can be inflexible in their routines and have significant problems with transition times, engage in some odd mannerisms such as hand flapping, spinning, etc. and sometimes have rituals such as lining things up. All of these unusual behaviors can translate to having difficulties coping in group situations both inside and outside the classroom. These clusters of unique characteristics often coupled with significant attention issues, anxiety with or without obsessive traits can cause major challenges for these children and their families, as well as major problems relating to others in a socially acceptable manner.

Treating ADHD appropriately in these individuals allows them the opportunity to be more receptive and focused and enables them to respond better to the strategies designed to improve their social awareness and decrease their anxiety. With proper emotional, social and academic support these individuals have the potential to do well in careers that showcase their talents and often end up in the engineering profession, or in the computer field. Many are professors in Universities; others are renowned musicians and inventors etc.

These brothers who came to my office over 15 years ago, clutching their toy tractors and talking non-stop about machinery and their pet rabbits, endured years of prejudice resulting from a lack of understanding, both at their school and in the community. They were bullied, ridiculed and thought to be mentally handicapped in spite of assessment in a clinic to the contrary. With the enormous emotional and social support they received from their parents and their years of home schooling, combined with medical treatment as well as learning about emotional attachment and communication skills from their beloved dogs, these boys emerged successful academically. They graduated as honour students in high school and took their places in college. Along the way they have made excellent gains socially and emotionally and are able to participate in youth groups and participate in college life.

A major turning point in their lives occurred when Concerta (long-acting mrthylphenidate) arrived on the market. Instead of experiencing the rollercoaster effect of the short-acting Ritalin, the smooth effect of Concerta with its gradually wearing off period changed their ability to cope in all situations, allowing them to be more flexible and in control. It also helped them to respond better to other medications prescribed to control their anxiety and depression.

Lessons learned

- I thank these boys and their family for the wonderful visits and for teaching me so much about Asperger's syndrome through different developmental stages of life.
- Triumph over adversity can occur in spite of all odds.

Last words

There are many more stories to share about so many children, teens and young adults with ADHD who have found fulfilling careers in different walks of life. With the arrival of recent long acting medications on the market, dramatic turnarounds have occurred in the lives of many ADHD individuals who previously have been poor responders to their medications. Hopefully, these few shared stories have helped illustrate that there is hope for everyone. Parents should never give up their quest to find the best possible solution for their child, teen or young adult with ADHD. It is never too late to help them. *Adolescents can triumph over trouble, tribulations and turbulence.* There is a road to success and happiness for every one of them; one has just to find it.

"GO nEIRIGH AN BOTHAIR LEAT."
Old Irish proverb meaning, "May the road rise to meet you."